HEALTHY GUT, HEALTHY LIFE

A Scientifically Proven Plan to Reverse Disease & Chronic Illness

NICOLE SPEAR

Healthy Gut, Healthy Life
A Scientifically Proven Plan for Reversing Disease & Chronic Illness

Copyright ©2017 by Nicole Spear
Wellness Ink Publishing: **www.WellnessInk.com**

ISBN: 978-1-988645-07-0 (paper)
ISBN: 978-1-988645-08-7 (ebook)

Contact:
Nicole Spear
Pure Life Health & Wellness, LLC
www.purelifehw.com
nicole@purelifehw.com

Printed in the United States of America
Cover: Cathi Stevenson
Illustrations: Elliot Lovegrove
Design: Streetlight Graphics

A Note to Readers
This book is for informational purposes only and is not intended as a substitute for the advice and care of your health provider. As with all health advice, please consult with a doctor to make sure this program is appropriate for your individual circumstances. The author and publisher expressly disclaim all responsibility for any adverse effects that may result from the use or application of the information contained in this book. References are provided for informational purposes only and do not constitute endorsement of any websites or other sources. Readers should be aware that the websites listed in this book may change.

DEDICATION

This book is dedicated to Dr. Nathan Morris, my mentor and friend, who first allowed me to see the beauty of functional medicine in health and healing, and who continually encourages me to learn and grow.

I also dedicate this book to the committed individuals who let me walk alongside them in healing their gut and helping them rediscover the gift of health. It is because of you that I continue to learn and serve others.

ACKNOWLEDGEMENTS

First and foremost, I want to thank my Lord and Savior, Jesus Christ, for giving me the passion and ability to serve others in health and healing. The more I learn about His amazing creation called the human body, the more humbled I am to be able to care for this marvelous handiwork.

I also want to give a special thanks to my brother and best friend, Jonathan, who has been my constant source of encouragement. You never fail to tell me I can do more than I think I can, and you inspire hope and vision.

My mom, Sherri, deserves more thanks than words can express. This book was only possible because of your sacrifice of time and your dedication to helping me edit and rewrite numerous portions so others can benefit from its message. I hope this book is an expression of your success as my best teacher in life. I also want to thank my dad, Kent, for his contributions in helping me learn how to publish a book and making this book look its best.

Finally, I want to thank all the doctors whose involvement and influence in my life have made me a lifelong learner and a better practitioner: Dr. Nathan Morris, Dr. Jonathan Brown, Dr. Ronald Grisanti, Dr. Sonia Rapaport, and Dr. Nikolas Hedberg.

TABLE OF CONTENTS

FOREWORD

OUR SOCIETY IS EXPERIENCING A sharp increase in the number of people who suffer from complex, chronic diseases such as diabetes, heart disease, cancer, and autoimmune disorders. Unfortunately, our medical system lacks many of the proper tools for preventing and treating complex, chronic disease effectively. There is an absence of training in using appropriate preventative strategies such as nutrition, diet, and exercise to treat and prevent these chronic illnesses.

Since a very large percent of our immune system is located in our digestive tract, supporting a person's gastrointestinal health is a key concept for achieving overall health and preventing disease. At the root of many chronic health issues is an imbalance of the intestinal microbiome. Getting the "gut bugs" back into proper balance is critical to our overall health, and especially the health of our immune system. These friendly gut bacteria are so crucial to our health that researchers have compared them to a newly recognized organ. The simplest way to jump-start your overall health is to pay attention to your gut.

Intestinal dysbiosis (an imbalance in the gut microbes) leads to many deadly disease states, including inflammatory bowel disease, obesity, diabetes, liver disease, heart disease, autoimmunity, mood disorders, and even cancer. Shortly after birth, we are colonized by more than 1,000 species of gut bacteria. We can influence our gut bacteria through choices such as vaginal delivery vs. Cesarean section and breast-feeding vs. bottle-feeding; our guts are also affected by antibiotic use, eating industrialized processed food, stress, chronic illness, and poor dietary choices—all have a profound impact on which bugs predominate. It is important to keep your microbiome happy to prevent serious disease. It literally could mean the difference between life and death.

A healthy microbiome starts with a whole food organic diet rich in plant foods, healthy fats (such as coconut, avocado, and olive oils), prebiotic fiber sources, nuts and seeds, probiotic-rich living foods, and a variety of colorful fruits and vegetables rich in phytonutrients and antioxidants.

My own journey through life-threatening illness was a powerful force in showing me the healing power of nutrition and functional medicine. At 25 years old, a diagnosis of breast cancer, followed by a harsh treatment regime of chemotherapy and radiation, left my body nearly destroyed. I studied the healing power of nutritious food and supplements extensively in order to experience complete healing and remission from both breast cancer and Crohn's disease. I began by making major changes in my own diet, eliminating gluten, dairy, and all processed foods and eating nutrient-dense options instead. I was taught the power of appropriate nutritional supplementation in restoring my health and energy and healing the inflammation in my gut. Now, after a relentless pursuit of personal healing, I am completely free of breast cancer and healed from Crohn's disease! I believe that the human body can regain its health if given the right tools… and Nicole's book will give you those tools.

Healthy Gut, Healthy Life is a timely resource for patients and practitioners alike. As a fellow functional medicine practitioner, nutrition expert, and avid researcher, Nicole skillfully and systematically deepens your understanding of the body's healing potential and offers proven strategies for healing the gut. Included are many helpful resources such as a menu plan, recipes, and shopping lists to assist you on your journey to better health.

I encourage you to take the challenge and replace your discouragement with hope for a life of renewed vitality and vigor.

Jill C. Carnahan, MD, ABFM, ABIHM, IFMCP

INTRODUCTION:
THE FOUNDATION

At the young age of 12, the world of natural health swept into my life like a storm. My mother, a critical care nurse, attended a weekend seminar on health and nutrition. Little did I know how this event would impact my future. My mom came home and began to fervently strip our cupboards of all familiar foods. She tossed out everything I knew and loved. Strange foods such as tofu and tempeh, whole grains, and lots of vegetables took the place of familiar favorites. I had just become acquainted with the kitchen and it was quickly becoming my best friend, but now that friendship was on trial. The baking of pies and cookies was exchanged for grinding wheat berries and kneading bread that often refused to rise. It was a transition from quick convenience foods to creating a health-conscious cuisine.

As with every new relationship, there was a period of adjustment. Soon, a whole new world of variety and flavor began to emerge. Unbeknownst to me, it was establishing a foundational appreciation for a healthy lifestyle of using food as medicine.

As my teen years progressed, our country life cultivated a love for gardening, nature, and the art of cooking—all of which were vital for understanding the healing potential of food and plants. My mom fostered my love for the sciences in my homeschool curriculum, and soon, my passion for natural healing was born. After graduating from college with my pre-med degree, I took a small detour away from my original passion and was swept up in the glamour of traditional medicine, encouraged to pursue medical school. Fortunately, life has a way of bringing obstacles and roadblocks to redirect you back to where you were meant to be. I soon realized traditional medicine offered very little real "health" and turned my attention back to the healing potential of natural foods, plants, and lifestyle changes.

I worked my way through graduate school to become a clinical nutritionist and discovered the emerging world of functional medicine. It seemed the perfect marriage between science and natural health. Moreover, it satisfied my desperate need to know the "whys" behind health and healing. Little did I know, it was (and continues to be) a revolutionary force in the practice of medicine. My confidence in using food to heal grew as I began teaching nutrition classes at a university and witnessed students whose health and lives were transformed by applying the principles they were learning each semester. After I began working with a functional medicine doctor, I observed the impact of nutrition and functional medicine on the lives of desperate patients who had spent thousands of dollars trying to get well, including traveling to various doctors, and who had lost hope that they would ever experience healing. I became fully convinced of the healing potential of the body when given the right resources.

Our bodies were never designed to be broken. They contain amazing, intricate, complex systems that can withstand immense amounts of insults—but as with everything, there are limits. Fortunately, that is not the end of the story. That same amazing body, when given the right tools to function correctly, can heal and repair itself. There is hope.

The problem lies in the fact that we have been brainwashed to believe a broken body will always be broken. Therefore, we Band-Aid the symptoms to make life manageable and come to believe we must be defined by our brokenness. But this is not health. This is not vitality. This is not life.

After traveling down the road of endless drugs and medical procedures, you may have become skeptical, beginning to consider alternatives as your last thread of hope for real health and life. You may have fumbled through the world of vitamins and minerals, herbs, and other healing modalities, but quickly become confused and overwhelmed by the smorgasbord of options.

Hurting people grasp for anything that offers hope. Through my family's journey with chronic Lyme disease, I have experienced the desperation and dilemmas caused by a misguided or misinformed medical community. I have witnessed family members become disillusioned as they exchanged fistfuls of medications for fistfuls of supplements. Experts have suggested sauna, electromagnetic therapy, ozone and oxygen treatments, high-dose IV vitamin therapy, functional neurology, and brain training as magical panaceas. I understand how this feels, and I want to assure you this is not how health is supposed to look.

Let's step back and reevaluate the situation. The anatomy and physiology of all humans are basically the same, although our genetics play different chords that create individual songs in each of us. No matter who you are, though, your immune system is where healing begins. The name of your condition doesn't matter, nor the degree to which your body is broken. The focus must be on a strong immune system, which is vital for repair.

Looking deeper, the immune system is housed in and nurtured by your gut. If your gut is unhealthy, your immune system will fail. And finally, at the most foundational level, the health of your gut is established by the food you eat. In this way, you really are what you eat. This is the foundation of your healing potential.

In writing this book, dear reader, my goal is to take you by the hand and to give you hope once again. Regardless of what health condition you face, or what healing modalities you have tried, I want to help you reestablish the foundation of your health. I won't offer vain promises of miraculous healing, but I *can* promise that if you supply your body with the right tools, it will do its best to give you the best life. Your body *wants* to heal. Often the waters are muddied with symptoms, supplements or drugs, diagnoses, test results, and attempted therapies. I want to help bring clarity to the issues you face by guiding you back to the basis for all health and giving directives to help you build a healthier gut and, therefore, a healthier life.

So—will you take this journey with me?

HOW TO NAVIGATE THE JOURNEY

Would you ever try to fix your car if you didn't know how a car works? Or would you attempt to fix a virus on your computer without a basic knowledge of computer software? Probably not. Similarly, a basic understanding of the gut is essential before we can begin the journey of fixing the gut and restoring your health. So please buckle your seat belt, turn on the ignition of learning, and put yourself in a comfortable gear so you can focus your attention on the road ahead.

Before you take off, let me give you a few directions. There are different routes to the same destination, and I don't want you to get hopelessly lost on a country road in the middle of a cornfield. Nor do I want you to feel like you need an honorary degree in nutrition and biology to complete your journey. To help you navigate, I want to lay out a few paths you can take and let you choose the route that best meets your needs.

This book is designed with four parts that comprehensively offer the most scenic and thorough route to understanding how your health is rooted in the gut, and how to fix it.

Part 1 explains WHAT the problem may be with your health and how the gut is part of that problem.

Part 2 explains WHY this plan offers a solution to various health problems, rooted in the gut.

Parts 3 and 4 offer a succinct dietary and nutraceutical plan with accompanying resources to give you practical ideas for HOW to heal your gut and improve your health.

Every traveler will benefit from reading Chapter 1 to understand the basic facts of the gut and how it functions. It is a short introduction into this foundational organ and how it influences your health.

From there, you'll need to decide what type of travel you prefer.

If you enjoy scouring the entire countryside with a long, scenic journey and multiple stops, I suggest you read this book cover to cover. Chapters 2 through 9 of Part 1 can be technical and dive into the nitty-gritty details of human physiology. This background is important for understanding why we must begin with the gut if we desire a healthy life; however, many people may find themselves frustrated and lost in a cornfield if they are not interested in the details.

If you prefer to drive past the scenic stops and just get to the destination, where you learn how to fix your gut, I suggest you begin with Chapter 10 and then move along into Part 2. Chapter 10 introduces the healing plan by addressing stress management. From there, we will learn how each food group heals or destroys the health of our gut.

If you prefer to skip the journey altogether and want to book a flight straight to your destination, I recommend you read Chapters 1 and 11, after which you can skip to Part 3 and begin applying the gut-healing plan. There is one caveat to this route: you may not learn some information necessary to customize your dietary plan and will need to stick closely to the menu I offer. It is designed for individuals who need a convenient meal and nutraceutical plan without the fuss of gourmet meals. You can substitute any of the recipes in Part 4, but without a background knowledge of healing versus damaging foods, you should rely solely on the recipes I offer.

Finally, each chapter ends with a summary, so you can skip around or just review the chapter summaries, if you like. You may decide to begin with one route and eventually recalibrate your GPS to another route. Regardless of what you decide to do, please don't get bogged down—enjoy the journey to a healthier life.

PART 1:

THE DETAILS OF GUT PHYSIOLOGY
WHAT IS THE PROBLEM?

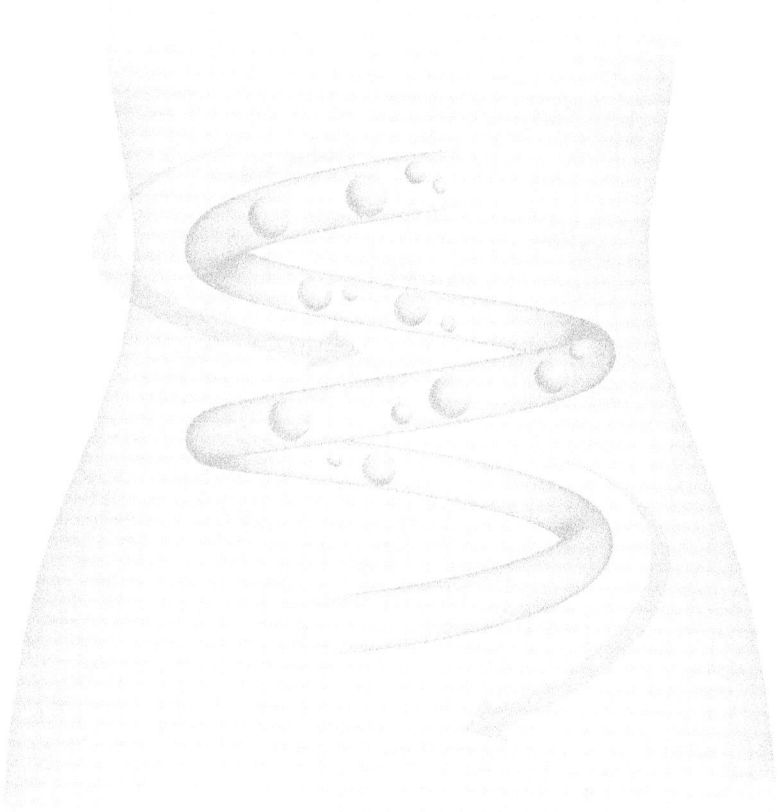

CHAPTER 1:

THE GUT

"All disease begins in the gut."

~Hippocrates, 400 BC

THE GUT DEFINED

M OST LIKELY, YOU KNOW YOUR gut as the digestive system. Quite simply, it is a self-contained, muscular tube that begins at your mouth (the gas cap) and ends at your anus (the exhaust pipe). The primary organs of your gut include your mouth, esophagus, stomach, small intestine, and large intestine.

The primary roles of your gut include digestion (breaking food into smaller particles), absorption, and elimination of waste products. Outside of these basic functions, it also participates in immune reactions, building hormones, brain function, and other bodily tasks. Some of these processes are complex, and all are vital to your health and continued existence. The efficiency of these processes can make your gut as streamlined as a Ferrari, or as clunky as your neighbor's old jalopy that probably needs to be donated to a better cause.

As food enters your mouth, digestion begins. From the mouth, it passes through a long tube called the esophagus, which separates your mouth from the acidic stomach. Digestion continues in your stomach, where the acid disinfects the contents before the food passes into the small intestine in a semi-liquid state. Nearly 90 percent of digestion occurs in the upper portion of this 20-foot-long tube. In the remainder of the small intestine, nutrients are absorbed and waste gets ushered into the 5-foot-long large intestine, which prepares it for elimination.

Several tight, rubber band-like gates that separate the different sections control the passage of food along this pathway. Waves of muscular contractions (a process known as peristalsis) allow the food to pass through the gates from one chamber to the next. Each chamber has a unique role in digestion.

The digestive system also includes four accessory organs responsible for producing and secreting digestive enzymes, similar to the chambers in your car engine that hold the oil, windshield washer fluid, and steering fluid. These organs are connected to the gut by ducts that open and close to release enzymes at the right times.

- **The salivary glands** in the mouth secrete saliva, digestive enzymes, and mucus as soon as our nose and brain communicate the expectation of eating.
- **The pancreas** saturates liquefied food entering the small intestine with a neutralizing bicarbonate solution and digestive enzymes.
- **The liver** makes a detergent-like solution called bile and stores it in the gallbladder.
- **The gallbladder** adds the premade bile to the food as it enters the small intestine; the enzymes in bile work to break food down and release essential nutrients that are absorbed into the body.

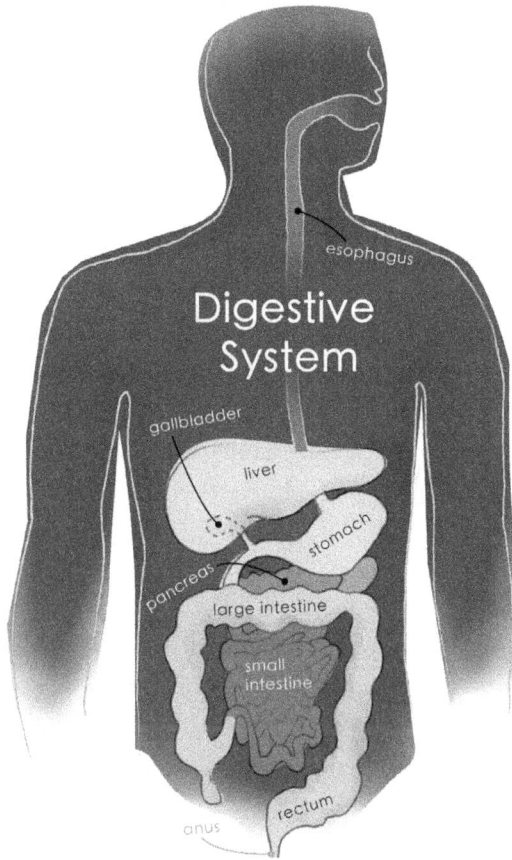

Digestive System

esophagus
gallbladder
liver
stomach
pancreas
large intestine
small intestine
rectum
anus

THE GUT AS A DOOR

The gut is to your body what the door is to your home. Every day, your gut withstands the abuse of harmful organisms, food-borne toxins such as preservatives and additives, dietary or environmental allergens, chemicals, and drugs. It attempts to protect your internal organs from danger by inspecting everything it encounters. It welcomes nourishing macronutrients, vitamins, minerals, and friendly bacteria, but it must be selective and astute to distinguish friend from foe.

It's easy to think that everything you swallow is absorbed into your body, but that isn't the case. Initially, everything is barred entry to your internal organs. Multitudes of healthy bacteria in the small intestine inspect the food, organisms, toxins, allergens, and other objects you swallow. They determine which contents are safe to pass through the small intestine and into the circulatory system, where the nutrients can interact with your internal organs such as the heart, brain, kidneys, lungs, and liver.

When the healthy bacteria in the gut identify potential dangers such as toxins, undigested food particles, harmful organisms, or allergens, they tag and usher them out for elimination. This protects the internal organs from dangerous substances.

The gut is like the door of your house because it stands between the external substances that enter the mouth and the vital organ systems of the body. It inspects and protects the body. Without the protection of the gut, the entire body would be exposed to any dangerous element we swallowed. Our bodies would be like an unprotected house without a door.

THE GUT IN ACTION

The unique architecture of the intestines highlights their role as a protector. Millions of cells line the intestines in unique fingerlike projections called villi. The arrangement of the villi increases the surface area of the intestines to maximize the efficiency of digestion and absorption. If the villi were unfolded and laid out flat, the surface area would cover an entire football field. However, the tiny folds are compressed into 25 feet of intestine, packed into your abdomen.

Billions of healthy bacteria coexist among the villi and secrete a thick, mucus layer, known as the mucosal gut barrier. It covers the villi, and protects and feeds its cells. The mucosal gut barrier also captures and inspects undigested food particles, toxins, allergens, and various organisms. Other functions of the mucosal gut barrier include:

- Helping to metabolize food,
- Generating certain B vitamins and vitamin K,
- Producing antibodies and enhancing the immune system,
- Generating antimicrobial compounds for pathogen eradication,

- Communicating with the brain regarding the gut's activity, and
- Manufacturing food for the intestinal cells.

Each villi encases a small vessel known as a lacteal. This vessel serves as a delivery vehicle for specialized packages of immune cells. The healthy bacteria communicate with these immune cells to combat the threatening substances captured in the mucus layer. Together, they inspect and eradicate the dangers. While this occurs, the cells of the villi are kept closed so the harmful substances don't enter the body.

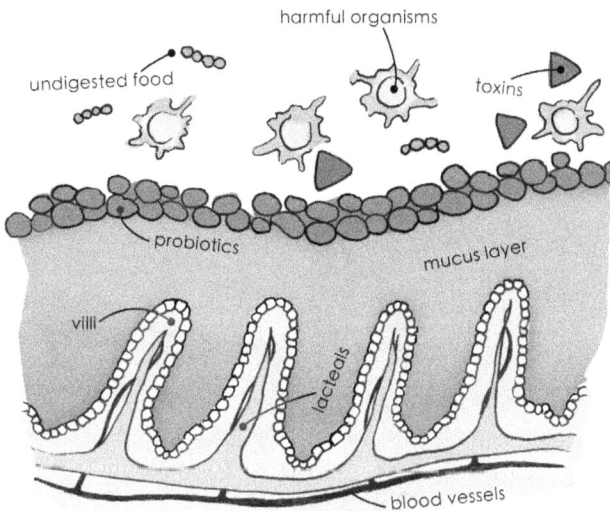

A Healthy Gut

THE DAMAGED GUT

The symbiotic relationship between the absorptive cells of the villi and the healthy bacteria in the mucosal gut barrier is crucial for a well-functioning gut. A poorly functioning gut jeopardizes the health of the entire body because vital organs are exposed to potential dangers. Weak bacteria can't secrete a protective mucus layer. Without this barrier, the cells are neither fed nor protected from the potentially harmful contents of the gut. Undigested food, harmful organisms, toxins, and allergens damage the cells of the villi and eventually destroy the entire structure. Once destroyed, the villi can't protect the body. The door is broken, and every organ system starts to suffer.

As our food becomes increasingly artificial, commercialized, and industrialized; our lifestyles more stressful; and the environment more toxic, our gut is exposed to an unprecedented amount of dangers. This hostile setting demands more security from the gut to ensure a well-protected body. But as our guts are increasingly damaged, they lose the ability to provide a safeguard.

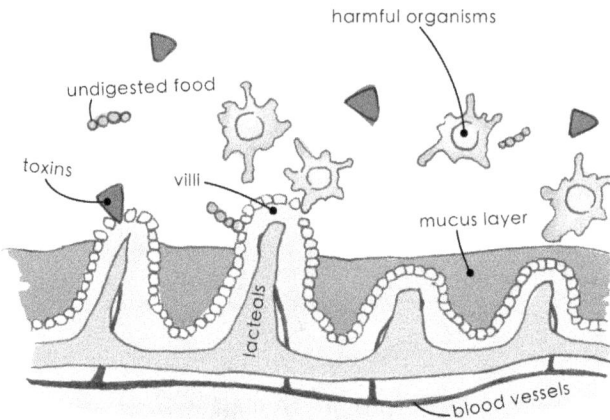

A Leaky Gut

Imagine finding a burglar in your home. Most likely, the routine tasks of the day such as the unfolded laundry, the unfinished meal, the dirty children, and the ringing phone are no longer a priority. Your focus shifts toward defending your home. The body works the same way. As dangerous invaders enter the body through a damaged gut, your body systems shout, "Code Red." All body systems divert their focus from routine tasks and remobilize to the scene of invasion. At this point, your health starts failing. Initially, you may only experience minor symptoms, but as the battle rages, you become increasingly burdened with signs of distress from various organ systems.

As the door of the body, the gut deserves your careful attention and consideration. If your health is failing, it's imperative to first examine the condition of your gut. Without doing so, we are trying to put out a fire while continuing to feed it with gasoline.

Chapter Summary: The gut is a self-contained tube that acts as the entry point into the body. It inspects all contents that move through it to ensure proper nourishment for all organ systems and to protect from foreign invaders. An unhealthy gut leaves the body exposed to dangers that threaten the health of our entire body. Failing health often indicates an unhealthy gut.

Key Points

- The gut includes the mouth, esophagus, stomach, small intestine, and large intestine.
- The primary roles of your gut include digestion (breaking food into smaller particles), absorption, and elimination of waste products.
- It also participates in immune activity, building hormones, and brain function.
- Fingerlike projections called villi line the small intestine and are responsible for absorbing nutrients and blocking invaders.
- The villi are protected and supported by a thick mucus layer, which contains healthy bacteria and immune cells.
- Harmful organisms, toxins, and allergens damage the villi, weakening the body's defenses.

CHAPTER 2:

THE NETWORK

F AR TOO OFTEN, THE GREATEST mistake we make when interpreting the nature of a chronic illness or poor health is to think of our body's organ systems as individualized compartments. If we focus all our attention on one to the exclusion of others, it is just as if we are placing all our eggs in one basket. We misunderstand the complex network of our body systems.

The inner workings of the body are often compared to a machine, and this is not by accident. Just as a machine or engine functions most efficiently with well-oiled and carefully maintained belts, bolts, shafts, and electrical systems, the body also works optimally when all systems are balanced. One worn belt or misfiring cylinder will place additional stress on the other components of the system. The gut functions in a similar fashion. When the function of the gut is compromised, all other organ systems struggle to perform. Body systems do not operate as independent entities.

Let's consider the primary organ systems of the body and their relationship to the gut.

NERVOUS SYSTEM

The nervous system, composed of the brain, spinal column, and nerves, is a critical component of our health and wellness and requires careful nutritional care. The brain alone consumes nearly 20 percent of the energy provided by the diet and is one of the few organs that demands a steady source of glucose for optimal functioning. It also requires a constant supply of essential vitamins and adequate protein to produce neurotransmitters (brain chemicals). The fatty neural tissue of this system is maintained by a good dose of healthy fats. Nearly every vitamin and mineral deficiency has been shown to impact the nervous system negatively.

The nervous system is adversely affected by modern food additives and preservatives. Tension, headaches, irritability, depression, and anxiety are common side effects of food colorings, monosodium glutamate, nitrites and nitrates, and various other artificial food toxins. In fact, therapists have often used nutritional therapies to treat certain brain conditions such as epilepsy, autism, schizophrenia, and ADHD. Nutrition undoubtedly impacts the nervous system.

The gut is often called the "little brain" of the body because it contains between 200 and 600 million neurons, which form the enteric (gut) nervous system. This specialized communication system is known as the gut-brain axis. The bacteria in the gut determine the number and function of these neurons, which send messages to the brain regarding gut motility, pain perception, abdominal distension, and transit time, among other activities.

The gut bacteria also produce neurotransmitters and compounds needed for neurotransmitter production. Neurotransmitters influence our mood, circadian rhythms, and behavior.

Gut bacteria impact the development of the central nervous system, memory, anxiety, depression, and the stress response.[1] Your behavior, memory, attention, and cognition are highly dependent on the intricate relationship between your gut bacteria and your brain.

SKELETAL SYSTEM

We are told that if you want to build strong bones, you should drink more milk, right? So why do so many of us suffer from degenerative bone conditions?

The hard material of bones acts as the body's storehouse for calcium and phosphorus. In addition to these major minerals, a healthy bone structure also depends on vitamins D, K, and C, magnesium, copper, zinc; and manganese. The availability of these nutrients is critical for good bone health, but just because they are in your food or supplements doesn't guarantee they are being absorbed and utilized by the skeletal system.

Lodged within the cells of the small intestine are multiple vitamin D receptors. A receptor is simply a mini-door that is specific for one or two nutrients. The vitamin D receptors in the gut use active vitamin D to usher calcium from the small intestine into the body.[2] When the body needs additional calcium, it is also possible for that mineral to slip between intestinal cells (known as tight junctions) and enter the body.[3] However, when the cells of the small intestine have been damaged, nutrient receptors may be missing or inactive. The absorption of calcium is greatly diminished, which eventually weakens the skeletal system.

The gut's regulation of the body's pH[a] influences skeletal health and integrity. When the body is slightly acidic, the bones help adjust the pH and bring the body to an alkaline state by releasing calcium into the blood. Calcium buffers the excess acid and rebalances the pH. If the body is continually in an acidic state (due to drugs, toxins, infection, or diet), the cells of the skeletal system continuously sacrifice bone to obtain calcium, resulting in a gradual weakening of the bone structure and density.

Maintaining an optimal blood pH is essential for preserving bone strength and integrity. A healthy gut supports this process by regulating electrolytes[b] (sodium, chloride, potassium, and phosphorus). As fluid and electrolytes flood the gut, specific transporters in the gut cells will control the amount of electrolytes absorbed into the body. When the gut is unhealthy, or when a particular gastrointestinal disorder is present, electrolyte balances are compromised, leading to pH imbalances that must be corrected by the skeletal system. Regular episodes of diarrhea or vomiting, routine use of laxatives, and chronic infections also lead to electrolyte imbalances and shifts in the body's pH, gradually affecting the health of the skeletal system.[4]

All body systems require balanced hormones to function at their best. In

---

a   pH is a measure of acidity. The pH scale ranges from a strong acid (pH = 0), to a strong base (pH = 14). A healthy blood pH is in the neutral range of 7.35 to 7.45

b   Electrolytes contain positive (+) and negative (-) charges. An imbalance of positive and negative changes will change the body's pH. An acidic pH occurs when there are too many positive charges, whereas a base pH will occur when there are too many negative electrolytes.

the case of the skeletal system, various hormones produced and regulated by activity in the gut communicate messages to the cells that are responsible for both building (osteoblasts) and destroying (osteoclasts) bone material. Serotonin, a hormone produced in the brain to help you sleep, is also made by cells in the gut to stimulate osteoclast activity.[5] Destroying bones may not seem like a good idea since we all want to build strong bones. However, every activity of the body must be balanced by an opposing activity, and regulating bone degeneration is just as important as controlling bone regeneration.

MUSCULAR SYSTEM

The connection between the gut and muscle health, known as the gut-muscle axis, is not a topic you will often find gracing the headlines of medical literature. Nevertheless, the connection is particularly important for individuals experiencing muscle wasting[c] because of a chronic condition such as cancer, chronic heart failure, chronic infection, or malnutrition.

Muscle is composed of protein fibers that can grow or deteriorate based on the demands and requirements of the body. When you use your muscles routinely or lift heavy loads, small injuries develop, stimulating the repair and growth of those fibers. This process is natural. Dietary protein provides the amino acids necessary to build muscle fibers.

Gut integrity and health is essential for adequate amino acid availability. When the gut lining is damaged, protein can't be digested into usable amino acids. If the cells of the gut are unable to absorb amino acids, we are left with a shortage that will impede muscle building. When the gut is unhealthy and damaged, consuming the correct amount of protein is futile since it can't be utilized by the body.

A damaged gut can also be "leaky," allowing undigested proteins to enter the bloodstream. The body recognizes individual amino acids, but not whole proteins. Large, undigested proteins trigger the immune system to shout, "Stranger!" and launch an attack against the protein. Therefore, a

---

c   Muscle wasting is also known as cachexia, a term most often heard in relation to cancer.

healthy gut is imperative for satisfactory protein digestion and absorption, which will prevent muscle wasting.[6]

INTEGUMENTARY SYSTEM

The integumentary system is composed of the skin, hair, and nails. Many common skin conditions, such as acne, psoriasis, and eczema, appear in conjunction with gut conditions because gut dysbiosis (imbalance of gut bacteria) leads to both local and systemic inflammation. As you might expect, various studies on individuals with acne have shown they are more likely to carry large amounts of harmful bacteria in their guts, coupled with insufficient amounts of healthy bacteria. Increased sensitivities to the toxins produced by harmful gut bacteria and other toxic substances cause systemic inflammation, leading to acne and various other forms of dermatitis.

Our skin is also affected by our ability to metabolize sugar. Gut dysbiosis causes problems with sugar metabolism leading to insulin resistance, which is perpetuated by poor dietary habits. As we continue to consume sugar, it fuels an unhealthy gut, leading to inflammatory skin complications such as acne.

CARDIOVASCULAR SYSTEM

Some say the key to a man's heart is through his stomach. While that might drum up images of candlelight dinners, sweet desserts, or a new charcoal grill, there is also a very real aspect to this cliché. The health of the gut contributes significantly to cardiovascular health, both directly and indirectly.

Diet is a key preventative measure in our battle against cardiovascular disease, the primary cause of mortality in the United States. Various diet-related conditions, including obesity, diabetes, metabolic syndrome, and dyslipidemia, have been identified as risk factors for cardiovascular disease because the pathology of each of these conditions involves the heart.

Systemic (whole body) inflammation characterizes all stages and forms of cardiovascular disease. As we will learn in Chapter 5, systemic inflammation begins in the gut. It contributes to the formation of atherosclerotic plaque and lesions, hardening of the blood vessels, and weakening of the heart muscle, which are primary contributors to cardiovascular disease.[7, 8, 9]

The role of beneficial gut bacteria in cardiovascular health is quickly becoming a topic of great interest within the medical literature. For example, high blood pressure is a known risk factor for cardiovascular disease and is moderated by gut bacteria. Certain strains of healthy bacteria, such as lactobacilli and bifidobacteria, produce compounds that are readily absorbed into the bloodstream and have been shown to have positive effects on blood pressure.

RESPIRATORY SYSTEM

In the gut-lung axis, the lungs function as an extension of the immune system. They encounter a vast number of airborne allergens and microbes and must identify and protect the body from invasion by harmful organisms.

Healthy gut bacteria influence all mucus barriers throughout the body, including the lungs. A protective mucus layer lines the lungs and acts as a barrier against environmental invaders. Its integrity and ability to perform its job well depends on the gut bacteria. Healthy gut bacteria promote optimal levels of immune cells in all mucosal barriers, including those of the lungs. A gut that has insufficient amounts of beneficial bacteria does not produce sufficient immune cells. In response, the body struggles to protect itself against invasive organisms.

Organisms that encounter the mucosal barrier of the respiratory system will eventually find their way to the gastrointestinal tract.[10] The gut bacteria identify harmful organisms and establish a healthy immune response to eradicate them. Once the immune response is activated, it sends immune cells to distant mucosal surfaces, such as the lungs and oral cavity, and establishes protection against the harmful microorganisms. Therefore, healthy gut bacteria are important for mounting a proper immune reaction in the lungs and protecting the body from respiratory illness.

ENDOCRINE SYSTEM

The connection between the gut and the endocrine system is highly complex and often overlooked. The endocrine system is the collection of glands responsible for secreting hormones[d] in the body. These hormones target specific cells and tissues, turning them on or off. Some of the glands of the endocrine system include the hypothalamus, pineal gland, pituitary gland, thyroid, adrenal glands, parathyroid, thymus, pancreas, ovaries, and testes. These glands produce hormones responsible for growth, development, reproduction, stress, homeostasis[e], and metabolism.[f] Problems within the endocrine system can have a tremendous impact on the health of the entire body since it acts as a master control center. Communication is critical for working together and, therefore, the endocrine system plays a crucial role in our overall health.

In the past four decades, the gut has been recognized as the largest endocrine gland in the body, known as the enteroendocrine system ("entero" means intestine). We don't often think of the gut as a gland, but it expresses more than 30 genes that supply instructions for producing more than 100 active hormones.[11, 12] The endocrine cells of the gut are located in the stomach, intestines, and pancreas. The gut bacteria also produce hormones that impact our health; therefore, these bacteria engage in endocrine functions.[13] The hormones they secrete are responsible for:

- fat storage
- appetite control and satiety
- production and secretion of digestive enzymes
- production and secretion of stomach acid
- production of insulin and glucagon to regulate blood sugar
- gallbladder action
- gut motility (movement)
- growth and repair of gut mucus
- fluid and electrolyte secretion
- inhibiting various enzymes

---

d   Hormones are chemical messengers that are secreted by glands and travel in the blood to other cells, relaying important messages about how cells and tissues should be behaving.

e   Homeostasis refers to balance and equilibrium among all body processes.

f   Metabolism refers to the collection of body processes necessary to maintain life.

- pain perception
- intestinal blood flow
- cell growth and differentiation
- nutrient absorption
- nutrient metabolism

As the largest endocrine system of the body, the gut is responsible for a well-functioning communication system that connects all our body systems and alters our health.

RENAL SYSTEM

The renal system focuses on the kidneys and their function in detoxification, elimination, electrolyte regulation, and hormone control. The kidneys also activate vitamin D, allowing enough calcium to be absorbed from the gut. They manipulate electrolytes and hormones to control blood pressure and heart function, which is why kidney disease and heart health are interconnected. The kidneys produce hormones that stimulate the bone marrow to make blood cells. Like all bodily systems, the renal system communicates with the gut, which governs its state of health.

Malnutrition, often stemming from an unhealthy gut, notably affects kidney function. Inadequate protein decreases the kidneys' ability to concentrate and acidify urine and eliminate toxins. Urea from protein digestion is essential for attracting and collecting water in the kidneys, thereby stimulating them to action and promoting detoxification.

Malnutrition may create an acidic body. The kidneys use the mineral phosphorus to capture excess acid and eliminate it to maintain a healthy pH. When dietary phosphorus is low, the body holds on to its supply, so it is no longer accessible to regulate pH, leading to a state of acidosis. As the body becomes more acidic, kidney stones may begin to form from excess uric acid. A healthy gut is vital for obtaining nutrients the kidneys need to maintain a healthy pH and prevent kidney stones.

HEPATIC SYSTEM

The hepatic system deals with our liver. The gut-liver axis is a well-established connection, and a consideration in many growing health concerns such as obesity-related liver disease (nonalcoholic fatty liver disease and nonalcoholic steatohepatitis), cirrhosis, and metabolic disorders.[14, 15] The liver is the hub of detoxification in the body. It is responsible for capturing, safely repackaging, and eliminating toxins. It is also a type of brain because it makes executive decisions regarding whether specific nutrients should be stored, delivered to another body system, or excreted. Since the liver has more than 500 functions in the body, it is an important administrative figure.

When our gut's natural defenses are broken, harmful organisms "leak" into the bloodstream. As unhealthy quantities of bacteria travel from the gut to the liver, they activate inflammation responses. Inflammation is a great instigator of liver diseases, contributing both to liver damage and the progression of chronic liver disease. Inflammatory cells in the liver can travel through the circulatory system, leading to systemic inflammation that destroys the gut. This cascade of events creates an internal storm that fosters continual damage to both the gut and the liver.

There is still a lot to learn about the gut-liver axis, but studies consistently show a connection between gut health and the progression of liver disease.

REPRODUCTIVE SYSTEM

Last, we will briefly look at the connection between gut health and reproduction. As sexual dysfunction and infertility rates increase, we are becoming more aware of the impact of diet and lifestyle habits on reproduction. The gut produces hormones that control appetite, satiety, and obesity. These same hormones also regulate sex hormones.[16] For example, leptin (which controls appetite) and insulin (which controls blood sugar) positively stimulate the hypothalamus to regulate healthy levels of sex hormones. Other gut hormones, including ghrelin (which controls hunger), inhibit the hypothalamus and negatively impact the production of sex hormones. Obesity changes the balance of gut hormones, which may explain the increased rates of infertility among obese individuals.

There are many associations between common reproductive disorders and gut health. Polycystic ovary syndrome (PCOS) is a common cause of infertility among younger women of childbearing age. High-sugar diets and insulin resistance impact the development of PCOS, as evidenced by the fact that a common drug used for type 2 diabetes, Metformin, significantly improves PCOS. Gut bacteria influence blood sugar regulation and insulin resistance and are therefore associated with PCOS.[17]

Endometriosis is another common reproductive problem connected to gut health. There are several species of bacteria in the gut that are capable of metabolizing estrogen and affecting the way our bodies receive estrogen. Therefore, gut bacteria influence estrogen-driven reproductive conditions such as endometriosis and certain cancers of the reproductive organs.[18]

Inflammation can have a significant impact on many bodily systems' ability to function at peak performance. The reproductive system is no different. It is sensitive to the effects of stress and inflammation that may be rooted in an unhealthy gut.

Chapter Summary: The body is a complex network of systems that function in unison. If one system fails, the entire machine suffers. The gut is a unifying organ among all the other systems, and if the gut is unhealthy, it weakens the health and function of the other systems.

Key Points

- The gut is the "little brain" containing 200 to 600 million neurons that build the enteric (gut) nervous system, as well as neurotransmitters that influence brain activity.

- The gut maintains a healthy skeletal system by regulating the absorption of bone-strengthening minerals, maintaining a healthy pH, and regulating bone regeneration.

- Through the gut-muscle axis, a healthy gut ensures sufficient amino acids are available to build muscle for strength.

- The gut maintains healthy skin by regulating inflammation and sugar metabolism.

- Diet, systemic inflammation, and gut bacteria influence the health of the heart and blood vessels.

- The protective mucus lining of the lungs is an extension of a healthy mucus barrier in the gut.

- The gut is the largest endocrine gland in the body, expressing more than 30 different hormone genes and influencing the production of all hormones in the body.

- The gut communicates with the kidneys to maintain adequate mineral supplies and a healthy pH.

- A healthy gut protects the liver from exposure to harmful organisms and toxins that may lead to liver disease and compromise its detoxification abilities.

- Gut bacteria affect the way our body receives and produces key reproductive hormones.

CHAPTER 3:

DIGESTION

"...bad digestion is the root of all evil."

~Hippocrates, 400 BC

T HE GUT MUST BE HEALTHY in order to carry out its own functions: namely, digestion, absorption, and elimination. The effectiveness of digestion is dependent on the production and function of various enzymes and the health of the villi.

Digestion, at the most basic level, is the process of breaking down large food molecules into smaller ones that can be easily absorbed and used by the body.

DISASSEMBLING CARBOHYDRATES, FATS, AND PROTEINS

Carbohydrates enter the body as large, circular strings of glucose molecules known as starch, or as highly organized squares of glucose molecules, known as fiber. The disorganized nature of starch allows digestive enzymes to enter the structure, break the bonds, and disassemble it into individual glucose molecules. These molecules enter the circulatory system and provide energy for the body. The organized nature of fiber, on the other hand, acts like a suit of armor, making the molecule impregnable by enzymes. These large, indigestible molecules serve purposes other than providing energy to the body.

Fat enters the body as strings of fatty acids connected to a head of glycerin. As it travels through the process of digestion, enzymes remove the glycerin head, while the fatty acid strings are captured and wrapped into capsules. Once absorbed, these capsules move through the circulatory system as the good "HDL" cholesterol, the bad "LDL" cholesterol, or as intermediates known as VLDL and IDL.

Protein digestion is not complicated, but the protein structure can be quite complex. Dietary proteins are long strings of amino acids tightly bound into a 3D shape. A protein may be made of a single string of amino acids, or up to four separate amino acid chains linked together. Peptide bonds hold the protein structure together. During digestion, digestive enzymes break the peptide bonds, releasing individual amino acids that are absorbed into the circulatory system and added to a pool of amino acids. Nearly every cell draws from this pool of amino acids to rebuild and repair tissue.

ENZYMES

Enzymes are the main players in digestion. They act as the solvent that disassembles protein, fats, and carbohydrates into their smallest parts. Our bodies contain thousands of enzymes with many functions, but the digestive enzymes are relatively easy to remember. They are named after their place of origin and the molecule they digest. For example, proteases digest protein. Lipases digest lipids (fats). And amylases digest carbohydrates (amylose is a type of sugar, a carbohydrate).

As soon as food enters your mouth, enzymes begin the process of digestion. Salivary amylase is the first enzyme on the scene. It targets the carbohydrates and starts to break down any starch into smaller glucose strands. However, food doesn't spend much time in the mouth, so the action of salivary amylase is limited. It is always a good idea to chew your food well so the salivary amylase has time to work.

As the food moves to the stomach, protein is targeted for digestion. Its structure is resilient and requires the highly acidic environment of the stomach to begin unfolding the tightly bound amino acid strings (a process known as denaturing). Protein remains in the stomach until it is adequately unfolded, paving the way for pancreatic proteases to finish the job of breaking the amino acid strings apart in the small intestine. If the cells of the stomach can't secrete sufficient amounts of hydrochloric acid, protein digestion will be impaired. Protein will then remain in the stomach, giving rise to increased air pressure, bloating, and acid reflux.

A small amount of gastric (stomach) lipase begins to digest dietary lipids in the stomach; however, most lipid digestion occurs in the next segment of the gut. Carbohydrates pass through the stomach almost entirely unnoticed, which explains why carbohydrates rarely make us feel full.

The stomach releases small amounts of its contents into the small intestine through the pyloric sphincter, a rubber band-like opening that controls the rate at which food passes through the digestive system. The passage through the small intestine is very similar to an automated car wash. Almost as soon as food enters the small intestine, the contents are identified and ducts on the sides of the intestinal walls begin to squirt a variety of chemicals and enzymes into the mixture. First, the pancreas squirts a hefty dose of neutralizing bicarbonate to protect the walls of the small intestine from the acidity of the stomach contents. Next, pancreatic amylase is added to continue digesting starch. The gallbladder adds bile to emulsify the fats, allowing pancreatic lipase to disassemble the fatty acids from their glycerol head. Pancreatic proteases finish breaking the peptide bonds between any connected amino acids that slipped in from the stomach.

As food molecules travel further into the small intestine, they encounter the mucosal gut barrier and the villi. Specific enzymes secreted by the villi complete the digestion of any remaining molecules missed by the pancreatic enzymes.

The enzymatic activity of the gut disassembles the original protein, fat, and carbohydrate molecules into building blocks of amino acids, fatty acids, and glucose. These small molecules can pass from the outside world through the body's security clearance station (the mucosal gut barrier) and into the body.

VITAMINS AND MINERALS

Glucose, fatty acids, and amino acids are essential macronutrients, needed in large quantities for hundreds of metabolic and anabolic processes. Vitamins and minerals, meanwhile, are micronutrients, required in small quantities. Every micronutrient undergoes a unique process by which it is absorbed from the small intestine into the body. Most vitamins and minerals are extracted from their food source by enzymes and then bound to a carrier molecule that transports them across the cells of the villi and into the bloodstream. Some vitamins and minerals can pass directly through the cells without assistance.

Most minerals are bound to molecules in food and must be repackaged before they can be absorbed. These repackaged minerals are called chelates. Some minerals have specific "carrier" receptors on the cells of the villi that recognize and transport them into the bloodstream. The body's mineral needs are always changing, and as it communicates those needs to the receptors, they adjust the amount of minerals allowed in.

Vitamins are classified as water-soluble or fat-soluble. Fat-soluble vitamins (vitamins A, D, K, and E) require bile to detach them from their food source, but they also need a fat-soluble transport molecule to carry them into the bloodstream. Needing a fat-soluble transporter slows the absorption of fat-soluble vitamins, so only 50 percent of all ingested fat-soluble vitamins get absorbed into the body.

Water-soluble vitamins (B-complex vitamins and vitamin C) are easily absorbed, but require larger supplies. Enzymes must be present to release the vitamins from the proteins they are bound to in food. Once released, they are ushered through the villi with transport systems unique for each water-soluble vitamin.

Chapter Summary: Good digestion is essential for delivering vital nutrients to the body. An unhealthy gut impairs digestion and blocks nutrient delivery to our bodies, impacting every other organ system.

Key Points

- Digestion is the process of breaking down large food molecules into smaller ones that can be absorbed by the body.

- Carbohydrates (starches) are digested into glucose molecules.

- Fats are digested into fatty acids.

- Proteins are digested into amino acids.

- Enzymes are the solvents that disassemble carbohydrate, fat, and protein molecules.

- Fat-soluble and water-soluble vitamins and minerals are extracted from food by enzymes and absorbed using "carrier" molecules.

CHAPTER 4:

IMMUNITY

THE LAST TIME YOU VISITED your doctor with cold or flu symptoms, did he or she ask you about your diet? Probably not. Most of us don't think about the impact our diet has on our immune system, which protects us from common illnesses. There is truth to the common cliché, "You are what you eat."

But this might seem like a rather far-fetched idea. If the answer was as simple as fixing the gut, why would we need a highly sophisticated medical system? As we begin to explore the connection between the gut and the immune system, and between the gut and the state of our general health, the serious claim implied by this common cliché will become clear.

Here's the reason your gut has such a significant impact on your health: it houses nearly 80 percent of the immune system. Therefore, if the gut is unhealthy, it will impair your immune system and the body will deviate from its objective to heal. This intimate relationship explains why a healthy gut is so important for a healthy life. It keeps your immune system strong and prevents us from becoming victims of poor health.

The immune system functions to protect the body from infections and toxins. At the beginning of this book, we compared the gut to the door of a house. The gut works to keep invaders out and protect the internal organ systems. This task would not be possible without the active participation of the immune system.

To gain a better understanding of how the immune system keeps us healthy, let's take a brief look at how it functions. There are two types of immunity: innate immunity and adaptive immunity.

INNATE IMMUNITY

Innate immunity represents the broadest type of immunity and forms most of our immune system. Every human is born with innate immunity. Its tools include protective tissues such as the skin and protective fluids such as tears, saliva, and mucus. Each of these tissues and substances acts as a barrier to prevent invaders from entering the body. The hydrochloric acid of the stomach is also part of the innate immune system because it kills harmful organisms before they proceed through the remainder of the gastrointestinal tract.

The innate immune system contains several specialized white blood cells including neutrophils, basophils, eosinophils, monocytes, and lymphocytes (B cells, T cells, and natural killer cells), as well as the proteins of the complement system. These cells identify foreign invaders and destroy them. Many work together in an assembly line, with each cell type accomplishing a particular task. The intruder gets passed between cells, which collectively work to destroy the invader. The innate immune system also identifies and destroys cells that aren't functioning correctly (i.e., cancer cells).

The health of your mother's gut and her immunity at the time of your birth determines the strength of your innate immune system.[19] The mucosal gut barrier is a critical component of the innate immune system. When a baby is in utero, its gut is sterile, and neither good nor bad bacteria exist there. The first dose of bacteria arrives as the baby passes through the vaginal canal during birth. If the mother's vaginal canal contains an abundant amount of beneficial bacteria, they will colonize in the baby's gut and begin forming the mucosal gut barrier. However, if the mother's vaginal canal contains yeast and harmful bacteria, these organisms will settle in the baby's gut and weaken the child's innate immunity. Infants born via Cesarean section lack beneficial bacteria and begin life with a weak immune system. Breast-feeding is another way babies obtain beneficial bacteria from their mothers and develop a strong innate immunity.

ADAPTIVE IMMUNITY

The adaptive immune system functions like a natural vaccine. It recognizes, destroys, and develops a memory of very specific organisms so it will be prepared with a defense if they meet again. Unlike innate immunity, which takes a shotgun approach and blasts all the bad guys, adaptive immunity is like a targeted missile aimed at a specific invader.

A newborn infant's adaptive immune system is very weak because its mother's body protected the infant from dangerous organisms in the womb. As the baby encounters germs, his or her innate immunity helps fight while the adaptive immunity takes a mug shot of these new organisms. In this way, the immune system adapts to commonly encountered organisms.

The adaptive immune system contains B cells, T cells, macrophages, and antibodies. Together, this unit engages in battle with foreigners. The T cells scout out the enemies and mark them with special chemicals. They then fall back and signal the other troops to start combat. Macrophages rush toward the enemy, surrounding and engulfing them. T cells hold some enemies hostage and present them to B cells, which take a mug shot that identifies them for future attacks. These mug shots are called antibodies, and act as "wanted" posters for recognizing hidden villains. The antibodies give the adaptive immune system permission to attack these enemies in the future, without requiring orders from the T cells. As the body encounters more enemies, the list of antibodies grows, and in this way, the adaptive immune system adapts to commonly encountered foreigners. The more offenders we present to it, the stronger it will grow.

Adaptive immunity explains why people in various regions of the globe have adapted to the pathogens common to their living environment. But when visitors arrive, they are susceptible to the pathogens responsible for regional diseases.

LYMPHATIC SYSTEM

As the innate and adaptive immune systems fight battles throughout the body, debris and casualties are left littering the battlefield. The lymphatic system is responsible for cleaning up the aftermath. It contains a network of vessels that flow throughout the body and act like the gutter on a house, collecting the battlefield debris and sweeping it away. These vessels carry lymph fluid loaded with an abundance of white blood cells called lymphocytes, which are part of the immune system. They deliver the war debris and casualties to lymph nodes, stationed in clusters throughout the body. The lymph nodes are pockets of concentrated immune cells that filter and restore the lymph fluid.

Remember how each of the villi of the small intestine contains a lymphatic vessel (lacteal) that delivers immune cells to the gut? As pathogens attempt to get absorbed through the villi, the immune cells destroy them before they can enter the circulatory system and make their way deep into the body.

GUT-ASSOCIATED LYMPHOID TISSUE (GALT)

You may be wondering how innate and adaptive immunity are connected to the gut. The mucosal gut barrier is part of the innate immune system that serves to protect the body against invaders. Everything we consume contains some amount of foreign matter. The mucosal gut barrier actively screens for microorganisms; drugs; environmental chemicals; toxins such as genetically modified organisms (GMOs); and foreign food toxins such as preservatives, additives, and colorings. Therefore, nearly 80 percent of the immune system exists in the gut—an essential element of our body's defenses.

Gut-associated lymphoid tissue (GALT) is the general term used to describe the parts of the lymphatic system associated specifically with the gut but independent of the lymphatic vessels (lacteals) in the villi. The main players of GALT include:

- **Peyer's patches**: Special cells, located in the valleys of the villi, where macrophages, dendritic cells, B cells, and T cells encounter antigens and destroy them.

- **Lamina propria lymphocytes**: A collection of B cells found in the villi.

- **Intraepithelial lymphocytes**: A group of immune cells located between the tight junctions of the cells of the villi.

Let's see how the structures of the immune system and gut are integrated.

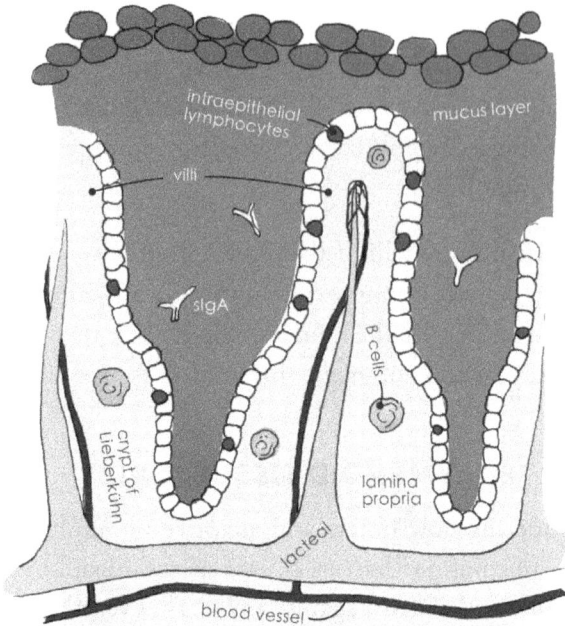

A Close-Up of Immunity

GUT MICROBIOTA

Now that we've gotten a basic overview of the parts of the immune system, we can turn our attention to the heart of the matter—the gut microbiota.

The human gut contains more than 100 trillion microbes, and the colon (large intestine) is estimated to contain nearly 70 percent of all microbes in the human body. The microbes within the gut are collectively known as the microbiota. As discussed earlier, the microbiota exists within the mucosal gut barrier and is responsible for metabolizing nutrients, communicating with other systems, and defending the host against toxins and dangerous microbes. This last responsibility requires significant participation from the immune system and, more specifically, the GALT.

The gut microbiota does dual duty because it must fight battles in the gut while evoking the appropriate help from the immune system. Busy communication is continually taking place between these two sides.

Imagine what might happen if there were insufficient quantities of beneficial bacteria in the mucosal gut barrier. It would be like an army missing soldiers. There is strength in numbers. Having an adequate quantity of beneficial bacteria in the gut will preserve the innate immune system. The troops in the gut are the front lines of defense. If they can take care of the enemy without requesting help from the innate immune system, they will do so. However, if their numbers are few and an enemy invades, they will immediately signal the innate immune system for assistance. In this situation, the body's internal immune system is continually active. An overtaxed immune system predisposes the body to autoimmune conditions and chronic inflammation, leading to other chronic health problems.

It's not only important to have sufficient quantities of beneficial bacteria, but also to possess the right *kind* of bacteria for a successful immune system. These organisms govern the state of both innate and adaptive immunity.[20] Your genetics, environmental factors, dietary habits, and exposure to infections and drugs influence the composition of your unique microbiota. This dynamic microbial system develops and stabilizes during your first year of life, but changes throughout your lifetime according to nutritional and environmental input. Even with your vast microbiotic diversity, two types of bacter*ia*—*Bacteroide*tes and *Firmicu*tes—should constitute a large percentage of every healthy gut.

Here's the good and bad news: your diet determines how many and what kind of bacteria reside in your gut. If you frequently indulge in foods loaded with sugar, flours, and grains and in processed foods, you will diminish your quantity of good bacteria. The good news is that you can regain the health of your gut by changing your diet. Parts 2, 3, and 4 of this book explain how to do this.

A PROBLEM: CHILDHOOD INFECTIONS

Sadly, immune problems can begin the day we take our first breath. Infant and childhood infections are so common we are becoming unconcerned with snotty noses, chronic ear infections, croupy coughs, and childhood fevers. Let's be honest, though: these aren't normal, nor are they indications of health. They're signs of a weak immune system rooted in an unhealthy gut.

An infant's gut is sterile until birth. While passing through the vaginal canal, the baby receives the same organisms that live in the mother's system. A healthy mother will pass along a good amount of beneficial bacteria to begin building the baby's defense system. Unfortunately, many mothers have unhealthy guts and weakened immune systems. Instead of receiving copious amounts of beneficial bacteria, the vaginal canal will deliver a dose of yeast and harmful bacteria to the infant. Therefore, many children are born with their defense systems already struggling.

When infants acquire yeast (*Candida albicans*) infections, they often manifest as cradle cap, oral thrush (a white coating on the tongue), fungal ear infections, and diaper rash.[21]

Occasional childhood infections are beneficial because they expose the child's adaptive immune system to foreign invaders so a memory of these enemies can be created to combat future exposure. But chronic childhood infections suggest serious problems. They are signs of a weak and exhausted immune system. As in any good army, rest and recovery are crucial for the success of future battles. When the immune system is continuously on active duty fighting infections, it becomes weakened and loses its effectiveness. Chronic treatment for childhood infections also causes serious problems for the immune system. Frequent doses of antibiotics or steroids destroy the gut microbiota and lead to long-term immune challenges.

A PROBLEM: ANTIBIOTICS AND CHRONIC INFECTIONS

So, what's the problem with antibiotics? After all, they remove the infection, right? Yes and no. They eliminate the immediate offender, but they open the door to other offenders in the aftermath of treatment.

To understand what happens to the gut after a course of antibiotics, we will use the analogy of a lawn treatment. Think of your gut as a lawn. Your lawn is full of weeds (bad bacteria, yeast, etc.). So you purchase a weed killer and spray your yard. Unfortunately, you were so anxious to get rid of the weeds, you doused your lawn in weed killer and killed your grass too. This same scenario occurs when you take antibiotics. They not only kill the problematic organisms (the weeds), but they also kill the beneficial bacteria (the grass). Now you are left with a dead, dirty plot of ground. If you ignore the ground, weeds will grow back and you're in even worse shape than before. This situation occurs in the gut, too. After a treatment of antibiotics, "bad" bacteria and yeast secure the opportunity to take up residence in the absence of beneficial bacteria. As they colonize, the innate immune system attempts to defend the gut, but without the help of the gut microbiota, it is overwhelmed and another infection begins. Once again, antibiotics enter the picture.

Do you see the dilemma? Routine antibiotics kill off the beneficial bacteria, allowing yeast and other invaders to colonize. The immune system becomes weak and chronic infections follow. This scenario is far too common among today's youth.

A PROBLEM: AUTOIMMUNITY

Another problem we face as a nation is a massive increase in autoimmune conditions. Some typical examples include:

- Type 1 diabetes
- Lupus
- Multiple sclerosis
- Myasthenia gravis
- Celiac disease
- Inflammatory bowel diseases
- Guillain-Barré syndrome
- Juvenile arthritis
- Some forms of anemia
- Psoriasis
- Rheumatoid arthritis
- Hashimoto's thyroiditis

An autoimmune condition is one in which the immune system begins attacking the body itself (as implied by the prefix "auto-"). It no longer appropriately identifies friend (your body) as opposed to foe (an invader), so it attacks both. For example, type 1 diabetes is an autoimmune condition in which the immune system attacks the cells of the pancreas. These cells are responsible for making the hormone insulin. When the pancreas is unable to make insulin, the body can't regulate its blood sugar levels.

Rheumatoid arthritis is an autoimmune condition in which the immune system attacks the joint tissue. As the joint tissue breaks down, the bones begin rubbing together, causing friction, pain, and inflammation.

In both examples, the immune system is overactive and confused.

Not too long ago, autoimmune conditions were considered rare. Today, though, nearly 50 million Americans are affected by one of approximately 100 different autoimmune conditions. Nearly 75 percent of these individuals are women. Chronic inflammation from an overworked immune system is the primary symptom associated with many of these conditions. Doctors control inflammation with steroids and immunosuppressants. Sadly, both treatment options have devastating long-term health effects.

There is a strong connection between the development of autoimmune conditions and your gut health. As we have been discussing, the immune system is built and nurtured in the context of the gut. If adequate quantities and types of beneficial bacteria are present, this first line of defense is healthy and protects the innate immune system. When your gut microbiota is weak or lacking, the innate immune system works harder to compensate. The stress of the demands weakens this delicate system over time.

The innate immune system can also become confused if the wrong types of bacteria are present in the gut. The correct bacteria communicate with the immune system to help it "learn" the difference between friend and foe. The presence of unfamiliar bacterial species silences that communication. As the immune system tries to function independently, both intestinal and systemic (whole body) autoimmunity issues can occur.[22]

Chapter Summary: The health of the gut is paramount in building a healthy immune system. An unhealthy gut lacks protective microbiota and exposes the entire body to chronic infections, leaving the immune system weakened and confused. This situation increases the chances of this system misidentifying invaders, leading to autoimmune conditions.

Key Points

- The gut houses 80 percent of the immune system.

- There are two types of immunity: innate and adaptive.

- The innate immune system is the broadest part of our immune system and is given to us at birth. It includes the mucosal gut barrier, as well as protective tissues (skin) and secretions (tears, hydrochloric acid in the stomach).

- The adaptive immune system develops as we are exposed to various organisms. It remembers previous encounters and protects us in the future.

- The lymphatic system is a network of vessels that carries immune cells throughout the entire body.

- Innate and adaptive immunity and the lymphatic system are present in the gut as the GALT (gut-associated lymphatic tissue).

- Gut bacteria preserve the mucosal gut barrier, the strength of the immune systems, and the health of the gut.

- Your diet influences the quantity and quality of the bacteria in your gut.

CHAPTER 5:

INFLAMMATION

W HEN MOST PEOPLE THINK OF inflammation, they immediately envision the reddened, painful, hot spot on a scraped knee. Or they think of a painfully pus-filled cut that won't heal. When I envision inflammation, I am transported back to my graduate-level pathophysiology course, in which I chanted "redness, heat, swelling, pain" for hours in preparation for an exam. You may not be aware of how inflammation can wreak havoc on all systems of your body. It is a root element of numerous health conditions, including cancer, arthritis, asthma, cardiovascular disease, acne, and even mental illness.

INFLAMMATION DEFINED

The medical definition of inflammation is "a localized physical condition in which part of the body becomes reddened, swollen, hot, and often painful, especially as a reaction to injury or infection." Although bothersome, this kind of inflammation is necessary for healing. It alerts us to the fact that the body is busy repairing tissue, cleaning up debris, and fighting off other opportunistic organisms that might be waiting to take advantage of the situation. We have all experienced this kind of inflammation, but there is a less obvious form of inflammation that is far more dangerous. Systemic (whole body) inflammation isn't always visible because it wages a war internally. This subtle battle secretly rages against all our organs and systems. And even more importantly, it begins in the gut.

The integrative and holistic medical paradigm recognizes that the process of continual internal inflammation acts like a metastasizing cancer, bankrupting the body's resources until it becomes weakened and overwhelmed. It is referred to as chronic, systemic, or low-grade inflammation. Its obscure nature makes it difficult to diagnose.

Chronic, systemic inflammation is the catalyst behind diseases such as:

- Chronic pain syndromes
- Obesity
- ADD/ADHD
- Autism
- Diabetes
- Cardiovascular disease
- Stroke
- Thyroid problems
- Crohn's disease
- Ulcerative colitis
- Cancer
- Allergies
- Asthma
- Anemia
- Alzheimer's disease
- Autoimmune conditions
- And much, much more!

This list may seem overwhelming, but the good news is that you can help control your body's inflammatory response through your diet and by maintaining a healthy gut. In Part 2, you will learn how, specifically, to decrease the inflammation that may be at the root of many of your health concerns.

INFLAMMATION IN ACTION

The immune system is responsible for initiating and maintaining a state of inflammation, whether localized or systemic. It uses special troops called the inflammatory factors (macrophages, cytokines, leukotrienes, etc.). Their job description includes launching and sustaining the inflammatory response. Here's a general picture of how it occurs:

1. The immune system alerts the body to potential danger.

   Foreign organisms, allergens, toxins, chemicals, injury, and trauma can trigger the immune system. Regardless of what triggers the alarm, the immune system immediately starts communicating with the body to spur joint efforts to remove the responsible agent and heal the damage.

2. The immune system directs inflammatory factors to the scene of danger.

   The white blood cells of the immune system are the initial responders. Being stationed within blood vessels, they can quickly arrive at the scene when an emergency rises. Once they arrive, they begin working while also secreting chemicals that attract inflammatory factors to the area.

   The cardiovascular system aids this transfer by widening the blood vessels for faster transport. The scene of destruction can get a bit crowded from the extra traffic and increased blood flow. To relieve some of the congestion, the blood vessels become permeable and allow excess fluid to drain away from the site.

3. While the white blood cells and inflammatory factors are busy working at the scene, the immune system communicates with the rest of the body via the central nervous system.

   It is important to get messages to the brain quickly, instructing it to induce a fever, increase fuel supplies (glucose) in the blood, and shift energy away from less important functions such as digestion and reproduction. These actions allow the body to divert more attention and resources toward healing the damage and restoring health.

In a perfect world, the healing process occurs quickly, bringing the body back to homeostasis (balance). After a brief episode, the immune system disengages and allows its troops of inflammatory factors to recuperate before the next event. This process is called acute inflammation, meaning it begins and ends quickly. It is a vital part of healing. However, as we alluded to earlier, these same processes can morph into a long, drawn-out performance. This new and dangerous situation is called chronic inflammation.

CHRONIC INFLAMMATION

When the body doesn't heal immediately, or the instigators of inflammation persist despite the body's best efforts, the immune system reevaluates the inflammatory response and changes tactics. It knows it must maintain a reserve of troops for emergency situations. It's also aware that the interrupted body processes need to resume.

To continue fighting the battle of chronic inflammation, the immune system changes its strategy and calls in reinforcements. Lymphocytes and macrophages remain indefinitely in the blood and at sites of injury or infection. If the inflammatory factors are working, the adaptive immune system is also in action, attempting to adapt to the crisis.

Danger mounts when these cellular activities persist for indeterminate lengths of time. This situation increases risks for autoimmune issues as the immune system wears down and begins to misfire, striking at its very own tissues. The danger escalates as the body strives to neutralize the constant stream of toxic chemicals released by the inflammatory factors to destroy offenders. The concentration of toxic chemicals can damage body tissues, leading to multiple health conditions.

INFLAMMATION BEGINS IN THE GUT

Chronic inflammation has become synonymous with systemic inflammation because as it lingers, it spreads throughout the entire body. Systemic inflammation almost always starts in the gut.[23] The gut encounters more potential infections, allergens, chemicals, and toxins than any other part of the body. For this reason, the immune system is highly concentrated in the gut.

In the previous chapter, we saw that nearly 80 percent of the immune system resides in the gut, operating as the GALT (gut-associated lymphoid tissue) in connection with the lymphatic system. Before toxins, chemicals, allergens, and infections encounter the immune system, they are filtered through the mucosal gut barrier. This barrier is laden with millions of beneficial bacteria and antibodies (sIgA) that act as the first line of defense against invaders. It also preserves the innate immune system (the macrophages housed deeper in the GALT) for bigger battles. If this first set of defenders is weak, then the GALT steps in to take action against the invaders.

Macrophages, the cells present in chronic inflammation, are located in the Peyer's patches of the GALT. They act as the second line of defense, following the mucosal gut barrier. They are responsible for battling invaders while alerting the rest of the immune system to an incoming attack. Macrophages are crucial for initiating chronic inflammation.

After encountering the invading bacteria, virus, fungus, chemical, parasite, or toxin, macrophages release special enzymes called cytokines. These not only target the offender but also alert neighboring immune cells to do the same. As the concentration of cytokines increases, larger players of the immune system rush to the scene. Cytokines are highly inflammatory and include the following chemicals:

- Interleukins (IL-4, IL-6, IL-12, etc.)

- Interferon gamma (IFN-γ)

- Tumor necrosis factor alpha (TNF-α)

Many of these chemicals generate free radicals, which are damaging atoms that assist in killing infections and allergens. The problem is that free radicals can also damage healthy cells. Therefore, after the cytokines eradicate the threat, another group of macrophages enters the scene and releases anti-inflammatory cytokines to block the action of the previous pro-inflammatory cytokines. They scrub the area of damaging chemicals, reducing free radicals and protecting the healthy cells. This cleaning action initiates tissue repair and healing, and all is well again. Of course, this tidy scenario is not always so neat. Sometimes the offenders remain and the battle continues, so the "cleanup crew" can't finish its job. Therefore, healing is postponed.

BAD GUT = CHRONIC INFLAMMATION

The strength of the immune system, and GALT in particular, is based on the quantity and quality of the beneficial bacteria and sIgA in the mucosal gut barrier. Having insufficient bacteria means calling the GALT to action more frequently. It also demands a stronger response, since the GALT must fight the offenders single-handedly rather than acting as a backup system that only attacks the larger invaders that escape the beneficial bacteria and sIgA.

When the gut is unhealthy, it lacks a strong mucosal gut barrier. The immune system is continually in demand. Chronic inflammation becomes a significant risk and soon creates a "leaky" gut.

LEAKY GUT

Many people have heard of the term "leaky gut." It seems to be a popular buzzword of the day. Leaky gut is certainly a topic of great importance among holistic health advocates, since it appears to be the link between the gut, chronic inflammation, and a myriad of health conditions. When Hippocrates boldly proclaimed all disease begins in the gut, he was recognizing a problem we are only now defining, two millennia later. That problem is leaky gut.

First, let's get a bird's-eye view of the process of creating a leaky gut.

1. Initially, the mucosal gut barrier either begins to lose beneficial bacteria or is overwhelmed by exposure to a significant number of offenders (food toxins, environmental chemicals, food allergens, microorganisms/infections, or stress hormones).

2. Because of the continual call to action, the mucosal gut barrier becomes weakened and thin and can't adequately protect the villi.

3. The GALT is forced into action, using its defensive strategies to engage the offenders.

4. The GALT communicates with the innate immune system to enlist inflammatory factors.

5. Inflammatory cytokines and free radicals damage the unprotected cells of the villi.

6. Damaged cells pull away from each other, breaking the tight junctions that bind them together and allowing the contents to leak out.

7. Food particles, microorganisms, and toxins begin leaking through the broken junctions and into the circulatory system.

8. These foreign objects begin to travel throughout the entire body, activating the innate and adaptive immune systems and resulting in chronic, systemic inflammation.

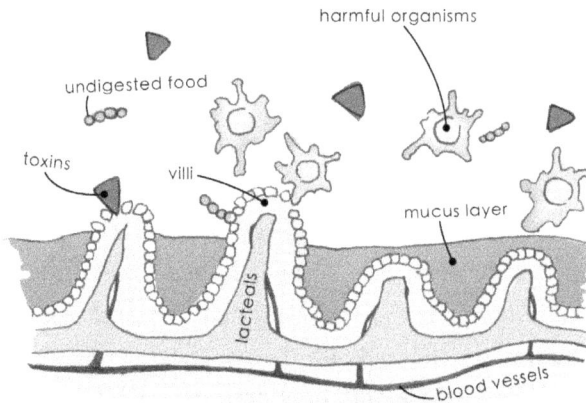

A Leaky Gut

Now that we understand how leaky gut develops, let's look at some instigators of this process. The causes are numerous, but these four are the most common.

Stress

When the body is under stress (either chronic or acute), cortisol—the primary stress hormone—surges through blood vessels. As it rushes through the blood vessels of the villi, it triggers the inflammatory response. If activated frequently or for an extended period of time, this response spurs the development of a leaky gut because it irritates the gut.

Gluten

Gluten has been a topic of much debate, provoking numerous passionate arguments from health advocates and practitioners. As we will learn later in this book, research shows that gluten promotes the secretion of an inflammatory protein called zonulin. It immediately causes the tight junctions between the cells of the villi to pull apart, forming a leaky gut.

High-Sugar/High-Carbohydrate Diets

Sugar feeds pathogenic bacteria, yeast, and other microbes in the gut, resupplying these enemies with ammunition. As these organisms flourish, they crowd out the beneficial bacteria, leading to a compromised mucosal gut barrier, activated immune system, and leaky gut.

Medications

Many drugs, and especially antibiotics, kill the beneficial bacteria in the gut, leaving behind an unprotected gut where yeast, infections, and toxins can thrive.

A compromised gut leads to a compromised body. A destroyed mucosal gut barrier and damaged villi leave gaping holes that allow invaders to wreak havoc on our bodies. This book began with the premise that the gut is the door to the body. A leaky gut opens the door and allows the enemies of health to enter.

The immune system attempts to mount a courageous attack, but as the battle continues, it becomes weak and chronic inflammation starts to threaten the body.

As we learned earlier, chronic inflammation is the underlying problem in most chronic health conditions. Let's focus on just a few of the most common conditions related to chronic inflammation, which begin with a leaky gut.

A PROBLEM: IBS, IBD (CROHN'S DISEASE, ULCERATIVE COLITIS)

Chronic inflammation in the gut is characteristic of both inflammatory bowel disease (IBD) and irritable bowel syndrome (IBS), although IBD exhibits more inflammation than IBS. Ulcerative colitis, which affects the colon in the form of many inflamed ulcers, or Crohn's disease, which involves widespread inflammation throughout the entire intestinal tract, are both forms of IBD. Gut permeability (i.e., leaky gut) and other structural changes in the mucosal gut barrier characterize IBD. Increased gut permeability activates the immune system, leading to diffuse and extreme inflammation in the gut.[24] With time, chronic inflammation leads the immune system to attack the gut microbiota and intestinal tissues.

IBS involves less inflammation than IBD but has a strong neurological component. Stress exacerbates both forms of IBS—constipation-predominant or diarrhea-predominant—because cortisol (the stress hormone) changes the permeability of the mucosal gut barrier, making it leaky and exacerbating inflammation.

Interestingly, both gut conditions—IBS and IBD—respond positively to probiotic supplementation, which confirms that the gut microbiota plays a significant role in the development of these conditions.[25] Insufficient beneficial bacteria, coupled with harmful organisms, lead to inflammation and a leaky gut, as seen in IBD and IBS.

A PROBLEM: CARDIOVASCULAR DISEASE

Cardiovascular disease remains one of the foremost health concerns today. This condition is also characterized by chronic, systemic inflammation, shown by high inflammatory markers on lab tests. As inflammatory factors (cytokines, interleukins, and other chemicals released by the immune system) surge through the bloodstream on a continuous basis, they damage blood vessels and weaken the heart muscle. Inflammation may begin in the gut, but a leaky gut opens the door to numerous threats that enter the circulatory system and travel to various locations around the body, causing further inflammation.

Inflammatory factors generate free radicals. These free radicals damage the cells of the blood vessels and destroy their integrity. The immune system attempts to patch up the damaged cells by signaling for more inflammatory factors. The vicious cycle continues.

Atherosclerosis also promotes inflammation in the blood vessels. Fatty plaques alert the immune system to damage in a vessel. The immune system calls inflammatory factors to the area to remove the enemy and promote healing. Unfortunately, while the macrophages of the immune system attempt to ingest the fatty plaque, they become enlarged and inflamed by the fat. The numerous inflamed macrophages and fatty plaque combine to form a messy jungle that contributes to more plaque development. Cardiovascular disease continues to progress.

High blood pressure damages the walls of the blood vessels because they must stiffen to withstand the pressure. This pressure damages the cells of the blood vessels, calling the immune system into action and initiating the inflammatory response. As the inflammatory factors attempt to repair the walls of the blood vessels, small fat particles floating through the blood vessels can get caught by the repair crew and plaque development begins. Therefore, inflammation caused by high blood pressure can lead to atherosclerosis and increase the risks of developing cardiovascular disease.[26]

A PROBLEM: CANCER

Cancer is one of the most feared diagnoses. Although the traditional medical establishment would have us believe there is no rhyme or reason for getting cancer beyond your genetics, a plethora of research contradicts this and proves diet and lifestyle choices influence your risk of getting cancer. Chronic inflammation is one of the most pronounced risk factors for developing cancer.[27] Cancer itself creates a state of acute inflammation. One way traditional medicine has combated this is with the use of NSAIDs (non-steroidal anti-inflammatory drugs). Although this is not the answer to this problem, it does prove the importance of decreasing inflammation when managing cancer.

Inflammatory factors generate a tremendous number of free radicals. They are used to kill invaders; however, when the concentration of these dangerous free radicals increases in the body, they damage healthy cells. Free radicals are skilled at dismantling a cell's outer membrane, gaining entry into the cell, and damaging the DNA within. DNA provides instructions for growth, reproduction, and all the cell's functions. Therefore, damaged DNA not only affects the cell's ability to work, but its life cycle.

Cancer, at the most basic level, is a cell that is growing uncontrollably.

Damaged DNA is one reason a cell might not be able to limit growth. Therefore, if inflammation can damage DNA, it can cause instability in a cell's life cycle, leading to cancer.

Chapter Summary: Inflammation is a response of the immune system to damage and infection. A destroyed mucosal gut barrier activates the GALT and initiates the inflammatory response at the area of injury or infection. As inflammation persists, the gut becomes leaky, opening the door of the body to invaders. These invaders systemically activate the immune system and a long battle rages throughout the entire body. Chronic inflammation ensues, and this is the root of nearly every chronic health condition.

Key Points

- Local inflammation is an immune response to a cut, scrape, or injury and involves redness, heat, swelling, and pain.

- Systemic inflammation activates the immune system throughout the entire body.

- The inflammatory response is carried out by inflammatory factors and white blood cells.

- As systemic inflammation persists and becomes chronic, the immune system is weakened and the body is at increased risk for disease.

- Systemic, chronic inflammation often begins in the gut because this organ houses most of the immune system and encounters numerous invaders.

- When the gut is unhealthy and leaky, a constant stream of toxins and invaders enters the body, which elicits an immune response and leads to systemic inflammation.

- Stress, gluten, a high-sugar/high-carb diet, and medications can all cause a leaky gut, leading to systemic inflammation.

CHAPTER 6:

INFECTIONS

I N THE LAST CHAPTER, WE defined the concept of a leaky gut and reviewed some of the most common causes, such as stress, gluten, high-sugar/high-carbohydrate diets, and medications. In this chapter, I want to focus on an often neglected, but very prominent cause of leaky gut—infections.

More people are infected with unfriendly organisms than we would like to imagine. One of the reasons this topic is so important is because many people attempt to jump on the bandwagon of health by cleaning up their diet, eliminating unhealthy beverages, and managing stress better, but they still experience bloating, pain, and fatigue. These cases are often due to an underlying infection that is interfering with full healing.

Sometimes, infections are the initial start of the downward spiral of ill health. Other times, an unhealthy gut leaves the body vulnerable to infections. So the train moves in both directions. Let's consider a typical scenario.

Sally gets strep throat, followed by bronchitis. The doctor orders an initial round of antibiotics for the strep throat. This is followed by a different antibiotic for bronchitis. After several rounds of antibiotics, Sally's throat feels better, but her gut's bacteria have been completely wiped out. Her gut is like an available piece of real estate, ready to be inhabited by the first buyer. Unless Sally replenishes her gut with probiotics that contain valuable bacteria, harmful bacteria and resistant yeast will seize the opportunity to claim the territory and establish their own clans. Although the GALT attempts to mount a defense against these unwelcome invaders, the ensuing battle only succeeds in damaging the mucosal gut barrier. Inflammation increases and, eventually, the gut begins to leak. In this state, the "door of the body" is open to other infections. Sally ends up wondering why she seems unable to stay well.

Let's investigate some of the most common infections that threaten the health of our gut and cause us to continually struggle with our health.

DYSBIOSIS

Dysbiosis is simply a new term for an old condition. It is usually heard in the context of leaky gut. You may already be familiar with this term.

We have been describing dysbiosis for several chapters now. It is a state of imbalanced bacteria in the gut. The balance between "good" and "bad" bacteria in the gut should always favor the good bacteria. In a state of dysbiosis, the bad bacteria are flourishing. When the bad bacteria reign in the gut, they become very dangerous to our general state of health. The mucosal gut barrier is ground zero for the battle between good and bad bacteria.

As we learned earlier, leaky gut puts the body at risk for multiple chronic health conditions and, most notably, IBS and IBD.

Strength is in the numbers if we are going to maintain the health of our guts. A thick mucus layer peppered with a plethora of beneficial bacteria keeps the gut in prime condition. If the native good bacteria are too scarce, the door is thrown open to a variety of unwanted guests.

There are many reasons for lacking healthy amounts of beneficial bacteria. Let's consider some of the more prominent causes.

1. Infants aren't gaining adequate probiotics or initial bacterial colonies from their mothers during birth because the mother doesn't possess a sufficient quantity of healthy bacteria, the baby is born via C-section, or is not breast-fed

2. Too much sugar or too many carbohydrates in the diet

3. Routine antibiotics

4. Chronic stress

5. Stealth infections (i.e., Lyme, Epstein-Barr, herpes, cytomegalovirus, etc.)

6. Exposure to toxins (food or environmental)

7. A weak immune system

8. Systemic inflammation

9. Allergenic foods

As beneficial bacteria are attacked or stressed by any of the above conditions, bad bacteria take control. Dysbiosis ensues and can lead to a variety of chronic health conditions.

SMALL INTESTINAL BACTERIA OVERGROWTH (SIBO)

This next infection is closely related to dysbiosis. In fact, the terms often get interchanged. However, these are two very different bacterial conditions.

First, let's look at the similarities. The infectious organisms in both dysbiosis and SIBO are the native bacteria residing in your gut. Both dysbiosis and SIBO create similar gut symptoms, making it difficult to decipher which condition is causing distress. Finally, both conditions, if left untreated, will lead to leaky gut and may evolve into IBS/IBD, autoimmunity issues, etc.

What sets apart SIBO from dysbiosis? Dysbiosis involves the overgrowth of harmful bacteria in the gut and can occur in both the small and the large intestine, but SIBO is a condition of the small intestine only. SIBO is an overgrowth of healthy bacteria that normally reside in the large intestine.

An abundance of beneficial bacteria may seem like a good situation. After all, haven't we been talking about all the reasons we lack these healthy creatures and why we need them so badly? But as we will soon discover, even too much of a good thing can be unhealthy.

SIBO is a condition in which the bacteria of the large intestine outgrow their natural habitat and begin to "spill over" into the small intestine. Upon entering this new environment, these bacteria are exposed to an entirely different food supply. The small intestine manages the digestion and absorption of nutrients, but the large intestine only accepts the indigestible parts of the food. Once the bacteria of the large intestine are offered the rich nutrient supply of the small intestine, they begin feasting and thriving in this new territory.

The bacteria responsible for causing SIBO love to feed on carbohydrates. As they eat, they release gaseous byproducts. Unfortunately, there is no place for these gases to escape. As they accumulate, you may notice a significant amount of belching, gas, bloating, belly distention, and acid reflux, with alternating constipation and diarrhea.

CANDIDA

Before dysbiosis and SIBO became so common, *Candida* was the hot topic. Cookbooks and anti-Candida diet plans quickly emerged, and it seemed everyone had *Candida*. Perhaps they did. Most likely, people were experiencing a combination of *Candida*, dysbiosis, and SIBO. These three infections often coexist and fuel one another.

How does this happen? Once one class of organisms invades the gut, it weakens the defenses so other unwanted organisms can also slip in, establishing successive infections. Eventually, the immune system is overwhelmed and can't gather enough troops to hold its lines. At that point, the floodgates open and the gut becomes prey to multiple organisms.

Candida is a fungal infection (yeast). Therefore, it has many characteristics that set it apart from the bacterial infections of dysbiosis and SIBO. It is more resilient, making it one of the most insidious villains in the gut. Unfortunately, this sly fungus is opportunistic, meaning it takes every opportunity to thrive. It easily crowds out beneficial bacteria and initiates dysbiosis. Maintaining a healthy diet and lifestyle is critical to containing this fungal threat.

Fungi such as *Candida* form "arms" called hyphae. Hyphae are like the runners of a strawberry plant. They burrow into tissues and mucus membranes to establish yeast colonies. When *Candida* is well established in a tissue, it begins to form a protective covering, known as a biofilm. This thick cover provides an excellent shelter from therapies targeted to kill the fungus. Biofilms make treatment tough.

The reproductive process of fungi heightens their resistance. To reproduce, they send out spores—spherical reproductive units encased in a hard outer shell. The exterior casing protects the spores from the immune system and enables them to travel anywhere in the body. They lodge in tissue and begin to form a new colony of *Candida*. As a result, *Candida* infections may start in the gut but can travel to the lungs, sinus cavities, vaginal canal, mouth, and other areas that provide a mucus bed for the spores to begin reproducing.

It is important to address *Candida* infections in the gut before they spread to other parts of the body, leading to chronic sinus infections, upper respiratory infections, vaginal yeast infections, and thrush (oral yeast). It is also important to contain yeast infections because they activate the immune system when the spores travel throughout the body.

Candida flourishes on a diet of sugar, dairy, and carbohydrates. Modern diets practically cater to *Candida* infections, explaining why they are so prominent. Yeast infections continuously supply the body with grocery lists, which the brain interprets as sugar cravings. That proverbial "sweet tooth" has a biochemical story behind it. There is no genetic predisposition at play, but rather, the presence of a yeast infection.

Candida is a problem for the gut because it fuels dysbiosis and inflammation. As it spreads throughout the body, it quickly becomes an enemy to our health.

PARASITES

Parasites include worms and other organisms that feed off their host (i.e., the human body). Once called "bloodsuckers," these organisms are repulsive invaders of the gut, and their presence is more widespread than we would like to believe.

Parasites physically damage intestinal cells, releasing destructive toxins in the process. The damage renders the gut unable to digest or absorb nutrients adequately. Malnourishment soon follows. Like bacteria and yeast, parasites weaken the gut's defense system, cause inflammation, and eventually impair the immune system.

Cryptosporidium parvum, giardia, cyclospora, and various families of worms are examples of common parasites. We contract these infections from contaminated food, water, or dirt. Some will cause immediate reactions; however, many accomplish their crime in the gut inconspicuously.

A healthy immune system (especially the GALT) and adequate supplies of probiotics and sIgA are imperative for fighting off parasitic infections. In the absence of these defense systems, parasites gladly take the opportunity to attack.

HELICOBACTER PYLORI

Helicobacter pylori is a parasitic bacteria that prefers to take up residence in the stomach. Most organisms are unable to survive in the acidic environment of the stomach, making *H. pylori* unique. It attaches to the stomach walls and uses its flagellum (a whiplike tail) to burrow deep into the thick mucus lining. It evokes an immune response that begins a cascade of inflammatory actions. Because of this cascade of events, *H. pylori* is linked to several health conditions, including:

• Gastritis

• Peptic ulcers

• Lymphoma (cancer of the lymph nodes)

• Gastric adenocarcinoma (cancer of the stomach)

• Gastroesophageal reflux disease (GERD)

H. pylori infections are becoming more common because of recent trends toward antacid abuse, including over-the-counter and pharmaceutical forms. Antacids neutralize stomach acid, making the environment more welcoming for bacteria such as *H. pylori*. Remember, hydrochloric acid is designed to kill dangerous organisms that enter the gut through contaminated food or dirt. Antacids cripple this important function when they neutralize the stomach acid. The entire gut becomes susceptible to infections such as *H. pylori*, dysbiosis, SIBO, yeast, and parasites.

STEALTH INFECTIONS: TICK-BORNE DISEASES AND BEYOND

So far we have looked at easily identifiable and relatively manageable infections. The immune system quickly recognizes them as invaders, and although they may initially dodge our notice, the immune system eventually alerts us to their presence.

Next, I would like to briefly look at another class of infections that is far more dangerous and even life-threatening. Sadly, these infections are becoming increasingly aggressive and common.

What kinds of infections am I referring to? Stealth infections. "Stealth" refers to organisms that can sneak into the body unnoticed by the immune system. They hide in our cells or masquerade as another organism, leaving the immune system confused or unaware of their existence. At this point, they begin to slowly take over many of our cells' normal functions and wreak havoc on our health. This process occurs subtly and results in generic symptoms, often misdiagnosed as chronic fatigue syndrome, fibromyalgia, multiple sclerosis, arthritis, Parkinson's disease, autism, allergies, hormonal imbalances, or other neurological and mental illnesses. Unsuccessful treatment plans cause more confusion and frustration in both the patient and the practitioner. Remember, stealth infections hide from the immune system, so detection is difficult, even by the most advanced test.

Stealth infections may include any of the following:

- *Chlamydia pneumoniae*
- Mycoplasma
- *Borrelia burgdorferi* (Lyme disease)
- Rocky Mountain spotted fever
- West Nile virus
- Epstein-Barr virus (mononucleosis)

- Cytomegalovirus
- Babesia
- Ehrlichia
- Bartonella
- Hepatitis viruses

Many of these organisms are tick-borne infections. Lyme disease is the most notable and is just beginning to gain public awareness. We will discuss the general effects of all stealth infections on gut health.

Poor gut health can predispose the body to stealth infections, but stealth infections can also disrupt gut health. We already know poor gut health causes weak immunity. Exposing a weak immune system to a stealth infection almost certainly ensures it will colonize the body. These infections gain entry through an unhealthy, inflamed, and leaky gut or through a tick bite or other vector. Once the infection enters the circulatory system, the weak immune system is unable to prevent it from spreading. Sadly, the infectious organisms seek shelter from nearby cells, where they reproduce and, later, make their grand attack on the body.

Stealth infections can also disrupt a healthy gut by provoking the immune system and generating inflammation. Therefore, they can be causes of dysbiosis, leaky gut, and other issues.

Stealth infections are experts at confounding our body's systems and disrupting biochemical pathways, hormones, and neurotransmitters. These outcomes make them difficult to diagnose and treat.

Aggressive antibiotic therapy is most often used to treat stealth infections. In severe cases, this is the only treatment option for gaining control over a life-threatening situation. We already know antibiotics dismantle the integrity of the gut. There is an unavoidable gamble between the benefits and risks of such treatment. *Candida* infections, dysbiosis, SIBO, leaky gut, and other gut complications are among the inevitable consequences of antibiotic therapy.

Some stealth infections directly cause dysfunction in the gut. For example,

Borrelia burgdorferi (the causative agent of Lyme disease), cytomegalovirus, Epstein-Barr virus, and herpes simplex virus cause gut paralysis (known as gastroparesis).[28] They penetrate the neurological system, disrupting the body's circuitry, and cause paralysis at various locations in the gut muscles. Inadequate muscle movement impairs digestion, absorption, and elimination, and allows ample opportunity for harmful bacteria and yeast to feed on slow-moving food.

Chapter Summary: Infectious organisms can destroy the health of the gut and promote the development of chronic health conditions. Healthy gut bacteria can outgrow their natural habitat, as occurs in SIBO. Harmful bacteria can gain precedence over beneficial bacteria, as occurs in dysbiosis. Stubborn yeast can take root and spread throughout the body. Parasites can steal nutrients. Stealth infections can be life-threatening. The consequences of these infections are inevitable and severe: poor gut health, inflammation, leaky gut, a weakened immune system, and the start of chronic health conditions.

Key Points

- Infections activate the immune system and initiate the inflammatory response.

- When infections persist in the gut, the inflammatory response damages the villi, opens the tight junctions between the cells of the villi, and causes leaky gut.

- Dysbiosis is an imbalance between the quantity of healthy and harmful bacteria in the gut. Dysbiosis progresses as the harmful bacteria grow more numerous and crowd out the healthy bacteria.

- SIBO is a condition in which the normal bacteria of the large intestine grow uncontrollably and spill into the small intestine, where they ferment sugar and create gas and bloating.

- *Candida* is a yeast normally present in small quantities in the gut, but when it flourishes, it crowds out healthy bacteria and spreads to other mucus membranes in the body, causing various symptoms.

- Parasites and worms initiate an inflammatory response and steal nutrients from the gut, eventually causing malnutrition.

- *Helicobacter pylori* are bacteria that burrow into the walls of the stomach and create ulcers and inflammation.

- Stealth infections are organisms that can sneak into the body, hide from the immune system, and masquerade as other organisms. They damage the body while confusing the immune system.

- Stealth infections are systemic and lead to a systemic inflammatory response, which can destroy the gut.

- A good quantity of healthy bacteria, sIgA, and other immune cells that build a strong mucosal gut barrier are important for preventing gut infections.

CHAPTER 7:

TOXINS

Toxins surround us every day. We breathe them in. We drink them. We eat them. We absorb them through our skin. We can't escape them. In fact, individuals carry such a significant toxin burden that the average infant is born with the residues of more than 200 toxins in the blood of their umbilical cord, reflecting their mom's toxin burden.[29]

Industrialization has increased the quantities and types of environmental chemicals we are exposed to regularly. Our bodies have the amazing ability to recognize, neutralize, and eliminate many of these toxins, but as our health declines and our exposure to toxins climbs, problems begin to emerge. Toxins start to accumulate in the body, where they disrupt biochemical processes, hormone balances, and the gut.

Consider some of the major toxins our bodies encounter daily:

- Herbicides
- Fungicides
- Insecticides/pesticides
- Disinfection agents (chloroform, bromoform)
- Heavy metals
- Perchlorate
- Phthalates (plastics)
- Phytoestrogens (estrogenic compounds)
- Polychlorinated biphenyls (PCBs)

- Polycyclic aromatic hydrocarbons (aerosols)

- Pharmaceutical drugs

- Volatile organic compounds (VOCs)

- Parabens (present in many body care products)

- Petroleum products

- Biotoxins (bacteria, viruses, yeast, parasites)

- Allergens (food, mold, dust, pollen)

Your genetics, in utero toxin exposure, the health of your detoxification organs, and your individual toxin exposure throughout life determines your "toxin threshold." This threshold is the preset amount of toxins your body can handle before becoming overwhelmed. As the toxin load in our bodies increases over our lifetime, we eventually meet this threshold. At this point, the body can't adequately process the toxins, and our health will start to suffer. Many people notice sudden allergies, sensitivities, and an inability to maintain the same level of health they once enjoyed.

Accumulated toxins disrupt the immune system, neurological system, endocrine system (hormones), and reproductive system. An overburdened body is a target for the development of many chronic health conditions. Our exposure to toxins is becoming a central area of research in the ever-growing cancer epidemic—especially among children.

THE GUT, A DETOXIFICATION ORGAN

The gut is one of the main organs of detoxification. It recognizes, neutralizes, and eliminates toxins. However, its effectiveness is highly dependent on having a strong, healthy mucosal gut barrier with an abundance of beneficial bacteria and antibodies (sIgA).

As toxins enter the gut, both sIgA and healthy bacteria recognize them as foreign and dangerous. The toxins get "tagged" by sIgA so cells of the immune system can remove them. Healthy bacteria will either neutralize the toxin or directly metabolize it into a safer form. A strong mucosal gut barrier serves as the first organ of detoxification, keeping toxins away from the body and preserving the detoxification functions of the liver.

Unfortunately, some toxins are readily absorbed despite the gut's best efforts to contain them. Pharmaceutical drugs are one example. Once absorbed, the liver must detoxify them. It gathers toxins from the blood and converts them into safer compounds. It then repackages the neutralized compounds and sends them to the gallbladder, where they are temporarily held along with bile. As the gallbladder squirts this bile into the gut, the repackaged toxins find themselves traveling through the small intestine once again.

Dietary fibers soak up the repackaged toxins and taxi them to the colon, where they are eliminated.

Adequate fiber is essential for detoxification. If the diet lacks fiber, the repackaged toxins can be reabsorbed and cycle through the body again.

TOXINS DESTROY THE GUT

Although the gut plays a crucial role in reducing your toxin load, it can be destroyed by the very toxins it attempts to eliminate. An abundance of toxins demands too many resources and overwhelms the capacity of the gut. Additionally, research shows us many specific toxins can disrupt the gut microbiota, causing dysbiosis and leaky gut syndrome. If the gut is leaky, the body's toxin burden quickly rises, since the preliminary detoxification organ is impaired. An unhealthy gut is the root of many chronic health illnesses because it can't protect the body from damaging toxins.

Let's review some of the most common toxins that affect our gut and our health.

PHARMACEUTICAL DRUGS

Let me begin with a disclosure. There are cases in which pharmaceutical drugs are necessary, and my goal is not to demonize them but to educate you on their impact on your gut. With this knowledge, you will be prepared to make necessary changes that will heal and protect your gut.

The gut microbiota recognizes pharmaceutical drugs as foreign substances that may be harmful to the body. The microbiota can't distinguish between prescription, over-the-counter, and street drugs. All classes of drugs are foreign and toxic as far as the body is concerned.

A healthy gut contains special types of bacteria that communicate with the liver so that it will produce the enzymes necessary to metabolize (break down) drugs immediately. Sustained levels of drugs damage the body. In fact, the liver is so aggressive about metabolizing medications that standard drug dosages are established according to the liver's ability to metabolize them. If the liver slowly metabolizes a drug, lower doses are prescribed, but if the liver quickly metabolizes a drug, higher or more frequent doses are necessary. The gut microbiota can up-regulate (increase) or down-regulate (decrease) the liver's enzymes. Therefore, a healthy gut influences the liver's ability to metabolize drugs.

Because many drugs change the gut microbiota, they can cause dysbiosis, leading to poor drug metabolism and an increased toxin burden, and can initiate the development of chronic health problems.[30]

Let's examine some classes of drugs that directly destroy the gut microbiota:

- **Proton-pump inhibitors (PPIs):** These are used to neutralize the stomach acid in those experiencing GERD (gastroesophageal reflux disease). Stomach acid is essential for killing dangerous organisms that enter our gut. Therefore, when PPIs neutralize the stomach acid, harmful bacteria are more likely to colonize in the gut. *Helicobacter pylori* is one type of bacteria that likes to grow when PPIs are used. As we learned in the previous chapter, *H. pylori* increases your risk for gastritis, peptic ulcers, and stomach cancer. The dangerous bacteria *Clostridium difficile* (*C. diff*) also flourishes when PPIs neutralize the stomach acid. These bacteria cause a potentially fatal form of diarrhea that leads to life-threatening dehydration in children, the elderly, and unhealthy individuals.

- **Antibiotics**: As discussed previously, antibiotics are notorious for initiating dysbiosis because they kill all forms of bacteria—good and bad. When the course of antibiotics is completed, harmful bacteria, yeast, and viruses are likely to colonize the newly cleansed gut unless you resupply it with probiotics.

- **Chemotherapeutic agents**: Gastrointestinal distress is a common side effect of chemotherapy treatment. The drugs induce inflammation in the gut and inhibit the growth of vital bacteria. Studies show chemotherapy drugs inhibit lactic acid bacteria and bifidobacteria, two classes of beneficial bacteria that maintain a strong mucosal gut barrier and immune system.[31]

- **Non-steroidal anti-inflammatory drugs (NSAIDs):** This class of drugs includes common over-the-counter pain remedies such as aspirin, Celebrex, Motrin, and Advil, as well as prescription-based opioids. NSAIDs are notorious for damaging the mucosal gut barrier and causing ulcers, erosions, and mild bleeding in the gut.[32] The gut microbiota also recognizes NSAIDs and alerts the immune system to initiate an inflammatory response. This may sound like a paradox, as these drugs are marketed to reduce systemic inflammation. However, if dysbiosis and SIBO are already established, the inflammatory response in the gut is heightened, causing leaky gut. NSAIDs enhance the damaging effects of dysbiosis. On the other hand, a healthy gut with many beneficial bacteria will reduce the gut-damaging effects of NSAIDs, although long-term use will still cause gut damage and ulceration.

As with many therapies, you must consider the risk versus benefit ratio. You are learning how gut health is a foundational element of whole body health; therefore, it is important to understand that pharmaceutical drugs pose a risk of damaging the "soul" of our health—the gut.

FOOD PRESERVATIVES AND ADDITIVES

The industrial era has supplied us with a plethora of conveniently packaged, highly processed foods. These food products contain preservatives and additives to extend shelf life and preserve texture and flavor; they offer time-saving food choices and easy options.

We may be led to believe these chemicals are safe, but the manufacturers know large amounts are dangerous to human health. Their presence in processed foods is acceptable on the premise that small quantities are not harmful to humans. Does this sound logical or healthy to you? If a lot of poison is dangerous, a little bit is safe, right? This logic deceives many of us. Processed foods don't come with a disclaimer telling you how much of their chemical additives are safe. Instead, the consumers who regularly eat processed foods are test subjects in an experiment that seeks to determine what level of food preservatives is harmful to our health.

Unfortunately, the damage done by food preservatives and additives is subtle and hard to recognize. It often masquerades as other health problems. Few of us realize the cost of chemical preservatives and additives on the health of our gut.

Let's look at a few examples of harmful, yet common preservatives and additives.

- **Emulsifiers:** This class of detergent-like chemicals improves food's texture and extends its shelf life. Some common food emulsifiers include Polysorbate 80, lecithin, carrageenan, polyglycerols, and gums. Studies show emulsifiers disturb the gut microbiota and can trigger dysbiosis, chronic inflammatory conditions, IBS/IBD, and obesity.[33]

- **Artificial sweeteners**: Aspartame, sucralose (Splenda), and saccharin are among the most common zero-calorie sweeteners. Nearly all diet and low-calorie foods and beverages contain these artificial sweeteners. Multiple studies provide evidence for the dangers these chemical pseudo-sweeteners inflict on our health. These artificial sweeteners induce significant dysbiosis, leading to gut inflammation and chronic health conditions. Alzheimer's disease, headaches, and even cancer may be outcomes of regular consumption of artificial sweeteners.[34]

PLASTICS

Plastic may be convenient, but its continuously changing chemical composition is a problem, as we're exposed to the harmful effects of its questionable constituents with no idea what's in the specific plastic we're using.

Major health problems arising from the use of Bisphenol A (BPA) led to its quick elimination from most plastics. Research shows BPA alters hormones and contributes to obesity. Unfortunately, BPA had been in plastic kitchenware, storage containers, and water bottles for decades before this discovery. As with many food preservatives, additives, and industrial chemicals, in the case of plastics, manufacturers are quick to introduce new chemical combinations into our food supply before adequate testing. Years or decades later, alarming studies lead to their removal, but not before they have done their damage.

BPA is still widely used in industrial manufacturing and found in the environment. As exposure to this chemical persists, BPA continues to disrupt our gut microbiota, promoting dysbiosis by inhibiting the growth of healthy bacteria. In fact, BPA influences the microbiota similarly to a high-sugar diet, which is a direct cause of dysbiosis.[35]

Despite the new explosion of BPA-free plastics, I would encourage you to be cautious with purchasing any plastic product. Plastic, by nature, is an industrial chemical. Glass, stone, and ceramic provide safer options for food storage and cookware, and years of use have proven they don't harm the gut.

PERSISTENT ORGANIC POLLUTANTS (POPs)

POPs are a group of industrial chemicals that persist in the environment and travel in both air and water. These compounds were utilized heavily in the early 20th century before we realized their harmful effects and took appropriate action to curb their production. Unfortunately, many are still in production, and most of us carry POP residues in our body tissues. POPs are among the 200 toxins identified in most infants' cord blood. The toxicity of these chemicals has been well established and linked to the high prevalence of cancer, as well as to neurologic, immunologic, and reproductive conditions.

POPs alter the composition, variety, and abundance of bacteria in the gut, making them targets for the increasing prevalence of gut-associated metabolic conditions such as obesity and diabetes.[36]

Let's review some common POPs that injure the health of our gut:

- **Polychlorobiphenyls (PCBs)**: PCBs are chemicals used in manufacturing electrical equipment, hydraulic systems, and other industrial materials. PCBs significantly alter the gut microbiota by decreasing the abundance of beneficial bacteria.[37] Interestingly, PCBs don't seem to alter the variety of bacteria as other chemicals can, but the elimination of good bacteria allows colonization by dangerous bacteria and yeast, leading to dysbiosis. PCBs manipulate the immune system and cause significant inflammation, which further exacerbates dysbiosis and leads to leaky gut.[38]

- **Pesticides**: In the past, we were primarily concerned with DDT and DDD, but today, there are a variety of pesticides in our environment that are toxic to the body. Pesticides exist in the air, water, soil, and many food products. From the apples we eat to the Roundup we spray on our garden, our constant exposure makes pesticides among the most dangerous toxins. Pesticides include herbicides, fungicides, insecticides, and antimicrobials. Seasonal bug spray, hand sanitizer, and lawn fertilizer all contain pesticides that threaten the health of our gut. The gut microbiota metabolizes many pesticides, allowing them access to our gut. Glyphosate (Roundup) promotes dysbiosis because beneficial bacteria are susceptible to damage by this herbicide. Harmful bacteria such as *Salmonella* and *Clostridium* are resistant to this pesticide and quickly grow in its presence.[39] Exposure to chlorpyrifos (a common insecticide used on vegetables) during pregnancy encourages dysbiosis throughout the infant's life.

HEAVY METALS

Heavy metals contaminate our air, water, and soil. Some foods such as rice and seafood can contribute to toxic levels of heavy metals in the human body. Mercury, lead, cadmium, and arsenic are among the most toxic.

Arsenic, recently discovered in rice and common in drinking water, is especially villainous in its actions against the gut. Not only does it change the composition of bacteria in the gut, but as microbiota metabolizes arsenic, those bacteria release other toxic byproducts. Often, these byproducts are more toxic than the heavy metal itself. Arsenic does a superb job of destroying *Firmicutes*, a beneficial gut bacterium that controls energy intake.[40] Having reduced levels of *Firmicutes* increases the risk of obesity.

Arsenic's ability to change both the composition and the activity of the gut microbiota establishes its connection to various health conditions including cancer, diabetes, and cardiovascular disease.[41]

AIR POLLUTION

Sadly, we no longer live in an environment where air is the clean, health-promoting substance it once was. Although vital for our existence, it is full of toxic chemicals that steal our quality of life.

Air is a carrier for volatile organic compounds (VOCs), combustion pollutants from fossil fuels, industrial chemicals, sulfates, pollen, nitrates, organic carbon, mineral dust, polycyclic aromatic hydrocarbons (PAHs), heavy metals, ions, and biological components. You aren't alone if you think this is a long list of foreign terms. The myriad of environmental toxins creates a language of its own, and unfortunately, the air we breathe transports thousands of these toxins to us.

The nasal hairs and mucus inside our nose captures small molecules of pollutants in the air. They are then transported to the gut, where the microbiota screens and identifies them as friend or foe. Those labeled as "toxic" are neutralized and eliminated. Routine exposure to air pollution like that found in urban cities increases the incidence of various gut diseases. As the microbiota strives to neutralize the air pollutants, they become overworked, and inflammation follows.[42]

Exposure to nitrogen dioxide has been linked to Crohn's disease in a dose-dependent manner, meaning the greater the exposure, the higher the risk. The total concentration of air pollutants is linked to IBD, and short-term air pollution is associated with gastrointestinal diseases. Ozone has been connected to appendicitis, while acute air pollution has sent several women to the emergency room with abdominal pain. Apparently, the air we breathe affects our gut.

These incidents point to alterations in the composition and the function of gut microbiota. Dysbiosis is inevitable, but another phenomenon occurs as well. When gut bacteria metabolize air pollutants, they release toxic compounds that react with each other and contribute to the development of several gut conditions. Gut bacteria damaged by pollutants can display altered behavior. They begin to ferment (eat) unnatural food sources and leave the gut void of the vital nutrients it needs to survive. A lack of nutrients destroys the mucosal gut barrier, establishes leaky gut, and weakens the immune system.

- **Volatile organic compounds (VOCs):** VOCs are making their debut in the public eye and, therefore, I want to bring your attention to this group of air pollutants. You may have noticed new paint and stain formulas sporting low-VOC claims. Hairsprays, aerosols, refrigerants, cleaning supplies, cigarette smoke, fuels, exhaust, and adhesives also deliver VOC residues to our body. Outgassing (the release of VOCs from materials that contain them) of many household products has increased awareness of VOCs and is partly responsible for the drive toward "green" living.

  Dangerous bacteria naturally produce VOCs when they ferment food. These VOCs cause IBD, some forms of diarrhea, and dysbiosis.[43] Using natural household cleaners and body care products, choosing eco-friendly building materials, and minimizing your exposure to paint and stain fumes will decrease your overall exposure to gut-wrenching VOCs.

Chapter Summary: As the first line of defense against toxins, the gut is particularly susceptible to the damage that can be conferred by toxic chemicals. When chronic health conditions persist and dysbiosis is a precipitating factor, it is important to evaluate your toxin threshold and strive to take the load off your gut by choosing to live as chemical-free as possible.

Key Points

- Healthy bacteria and sIgA, residing in a strong mucosal gut barrier, are responsible for neutralizing the toxins that enter the gut, preventing them from harming the body.

- Many pharmaceutical drugs including antacids, antibiotics, chemotherapy, and pain medications either destroy healthy bacteria or promote the growth of harmful bacteria, causing dysbiosis and leaky gut.

- Food additives and preservatives disturb the bacteria in the gut and are consumed in greater quantities than we may realize, as we obtain them cumulatively in common food products.

- Plastics often contain dangerous chemicals such as BPA that are known to disrupt the bacteria in the gut and cause leaky gut.

- Persistent organic pollutants such as pesticides and PCBs are persistent industrial chemicals in our environment, known to contribute to dysbiosis.

- Heavy metals such as arsenic, lead, and mercury are found in our land, water, and air; therefore, the residues of these heavy metals are in many foods. Heavy metals can change the types of bacteria that grow in the gut.

- Air contains numerous pollutants such as VOCs and polyhydrocarbons that can initiate inflammatory responses, destroy the mucosal gut barrier, and burden the detoxification ability of the gut.

CHAPTER 8:

THE GUT-BRAIN AXIS

I MAGINE THE FEELING YOU EXPERIENCE just before you step out onto a stage to deliver a speech or performance. Or the feeling you get before meeting a significant person. Perhaps it is the feeling you had when you walked down the aisle on your wedding day. These situations probably elicit memories of "butterflies in the stomach" or a "knotted-up stomach." Fear is a powerful emotion that can suddenly trigger a rush for the restroom, too. (Funny, you didn't need it a minute earlier.) IBS sufferers are keenly aware of the connection between mental stress and embarrassing reactions of the gut. In all these situations, the brain rouses the gut, and this alliance is one of the most underestimated in health.

The gut is known as the second brain. It may not think, reason, feel, or make decisions, but it influences your brain's ability to think, reason, feel, and make decisions. The gut affects the brain's development and how it functions. This relationship becomes more apparent as we discover a gastrointestinal component in a multitude of psychiatric and neurological conditions. As we will learn, ADD/ADHD, autism, depression, anxiety, schizophrenia, Parkinson's disease, Alzheimer's disease, and many others are directly related to the health of your gut.

THE VAGUS NERVE

The gut microbiota communicates with the brain through a central communication line called the vagus nerve. One end of the vagus nerve is connected to the enteric nervous system of the gut. This independent nervous system intricately weaves its mesh-like neurons through the mucosal gut barrier and the muscles of the gut. It controls the movement of the muscles, secretion of digestive enzymes, and produces many of the same neurotransmitters found in the brain. The gut contains 500 million neurons and the brain contains 100 billion neurons. At the other end of the vagus nerve is the central nervous system, directing all messages to its central processing system—the brain.

THE BLOOD-BRAIN BARRIER (BBB)

The vagus nerve isn't the only connection between the brain and the gut. The circulatory system also joins these two organ systems. The nutrients digested and absorbed through the gut are distributed to the brain by the circulatory system. The brain utilizes nearly 20 percent of all the nutrients we consume. As the blood travels toward the brain, the edges of the small blood vessels become lined with extremely tight cells known as tight junctions. Collectively, they form the blood-brain barrier (BBB). This layer of tight cells provides extra protection between the contents of the blood and the brain. It is designed to ensure the safety of the brain by reassessing the nutrients or components that cross through it. Much like the mucosal gut barrier ensures our protection from dangerous toxins and microbes entering our blood, the BBB similarly protects the central nervous system from harmful substances. When the mucosal gut barrier suffers damage, the BBB must be more vigilant.

MICROBIOTA AND THE BBB

The presence of an active, healthy mucosal gut barrier influences the health of the BBB. When you lack an adequate gut microbiota, the tight junctions of the BBB loosen, allowing dangerous compounds and microbes access to the brain.[44]

Beneficial bacteria in the gut consume nutrients and release specific compounds called short-chain fatty acids (SCFAs). These are vital for keeping the villi of the small intestine robust and healthy by maintaining tight junctions between the cells of the villi. In essence, SCFAs prevent the gut from becoming leaky.

SCFAs also travel to the BBB and establish tight junctions between the cells.

Therefore, the gut microbiota produces compounds that not only maintain a strong gut barrier, but a strong brain barrier as well. SCFAs are like the ammunition for these two lines of defense. Without the ammunition, the defense is inactive.

MICROBIOTA PRODUCE NEUROTRANSMITTERS

Neurotransmitters are chemicals that control the activities of the brain. Some neurotransmitters are excitatory and create activity in the brain. Others are inhibitory and pacify activity to calm us and promote relaxation. Still others can play both roles, depending on the need. The balance of these neurotransmitters influences our mood, actions, decisions, and cognitive abilities. Here are some of the most common neurotransmitters and their functions:

- **Acetylcholine**: wakefulness, attention, learning, emotion, memory, muscle movement
- **Serotonin**: appetite, alertness, concentration, body temperature, emotion, sleep, pain
- **Histamine**: wakefulness, attention, energy, learning, memory, sleep
- **Dopamine**: motivation, excitement, memory, mood, positive reinforcement
- **Noradrenaline**: anxiety, wakefulness, sleep, memory, respiration, negative emotions
- **GABA**: Eating, sleeping, aggression

Many neurotransmitters are produced directly by neurons; however, a healthy gut microbiota can also produce neurotransmitters, which can signal the brain through the vagus nerve. GABA, serotonin, norepinephrine, dopamine, acetylcholine, and melatonin are generated by the gut microbiota to alter gut function. As they work on the gut, they also modify brain function.[45, 46]

THE PROBLEM: ANXIETY, DEPRESSION, AND MOODS

It appears that "gut feelings" are legitimate after all. In a very literal sense, our gut microbiota influences our feelings and emotions. Anxiety and depression have been the focus of many researchers, who are discovering several pathways through which harmful bacteria in the gut promote anxiety and depression. A healthy microbiota produces GABA, which communicates with the brain via the vagus nerve. GABA is a calming neurotransmitter, and when it is lacking, we feel anxious, uptight, and stressed. When we lack adequate quantities of beneficial bacteria, our GABA production is inadequate. There is a strong connection between dysbiosis-related gut conditions such as IBS and IBD, and mood issues such as anxiety and depression.[47] This association seems to be rooted in a weak microbiota that is unable to produce sufficient GABA. As we will see in the next chapter, stressful circumstances alter the gut microbiota unfavorably, creating dysbiosis, anxiety, and depression.

THE PROBLEM: ADD/ADHD AND AUTISM SPECTRUM DISORDERS

Researchers and holistic doctors suspected a connection between the gut and ADD/ADHD long before the literature began to support the idea.[48] Today, it is common to see food allergies, eczema, and other gut-associated problems in children with attention and hyperactivity disorders. In most cases, addressing the gut and allergy issues significantly improves concentration and decreases hyperactivity.

Autism spectrum disorders often respond positively to improvements in gut microbiota.[49] Inflammation and autoimmunity are often elements of autism. As we have learned, dysbiosis, leaky gut, and systemic inflammation are like a three-legged stool. If left untreated, this trio often leads to autoimmunity issues. Nearly 30 percent of all children with autism have a confused immune system that is attacking parts of the brain.[50]

Many ADD/ADHD and autistic children also have leaky guts that allow dangerous organisms, food allergens, and toxins to cross into the circulatory system. These potential threats travel to the brain where they meet the BBB. If the BBB is healthy, they shouldn't be able to gain access to the brain, but we know the gut microbiota influences the permeability of the

BBB. A child with leaky gut will have a weak BBB that may allow these foreign invaders to pass into the brain.

Harmful bacteria and yeast, most often associated with dysbiosis and leaky gut, can release toxic compounds that travel to the brain, cross the BBB, and exacerbate ADD/ADHD and autistic symptoms. For example, when yeast ferments carbohydrates and sugars, it releases alcohol and acetaldehyde. These compounds can cross the BBB and damage the brain and nervous system. Aggression, behavioral abnormalities, learning challenges, memory lapses, and speech impairment are signs of a brain damaged by alcohol.

Many children with ADD/ADHD and autism spectrum disorder are allergic to dairy and gluten (the protein found in wheat, rye, and barley). When these foods don't get adequately digested because of a leaky gut, large molecules enter the body and travel to the brain. These molecules can attach to pain receptors and act like opiates (drugs used to control pain) to block certain functions of the brain. This activity explains why dairy and gluten commonly trigger ADD/ADHD and autistic behaviors.

THE PROBLEM: PARKINSON'S AND ALZHEIMER'S DISEASE

An unhealthy gut seems to contribute to the development of neurodegenerative diseases such as Parkinson's and Alzheimer's disease. Parkinson's disease is characterized by "plaques" and "tangles" found in the brain. These anomalies shut down cells, reduce certain neurotransmitters (specifically dopamine), and affect muscle function and movement. Interestingly, the same plaques and tangles exist in the enteric nervous system. Several studies suggest they may start in the gut and travel to the brain, where they develop into Alzheimer's disease.[51]

Nearly 80 percent of individuals with Parkinson's disease have accompanying gut issues. [52]The characteristic plaques and tangles of Parkinson's disease create a loss of dopamine in the gut. Low dopamine causes poor gut movement and poor digestion, and activates the immune system. Interestingly, poor gut health often precedes the initial symptoms of Parkinson's disease, supporting the idea that this neurodegenerative disease may be rooted in the gut.[53] Finally, systemic inflammation, an outcome of dysbiosis, is present in all neurodegenerative conditions, including Parkinson's and Alzheimer's disease.

Like Parkinson's disease, Alzheimer's disease involves the development and accumulation of plaques on the neurons. Unlike Parkinson's disease, the plaques of Alzheimer's disease affect the region of the brain responsible for memory, leading to progressive memory loss. The plaques contain a protein normally present in the gut and used by the enteric nervous system. This protein is responsible for gut movement and helps establish a healthy immune system in the gut. An accumulation of this protein (characteristic of Alzheimer's disease) signifies a loss of enteric neurons and increased gut inflammation. Therefore, it is possible that an unhealthy gut could contribute to an accumulation of the protein, leading to the plaques that characterize Alzheimer's disease.[54] Researchers are still confirming this hypothesis, but if proved to be true, it would unequivocally link Alzheimer's disease to the gut. In the meantime, it is safe to say that systemic inflammation, originating from gut dysbiosis, is indeed associated with the progression of Alzheimer's disease.

Chapter Summary: The health of the gut influences the health of the brain through various avenues. The vagus nerve acts as a direct line of communication between these two systems. Messages that pass between them can influence our mood and contribute to anxiety and depression. The gut microbiota also influences the health of the tight junctions of the blood-brain barrier (BBB). If toxic compounds pass through this line of defense, they can trigger ADD/ADHD and autism spectrum disorders. Finally, the enteric nervous system can be a breeding ground for plaques associated with Parkinson's and Alzheimer's disease.

Key Points

- The gut is known as the second brain and contains more than 500 million neurons that make up the enteric nervous system. This system is connected to the brain by the vagus nerve.

- The gut is also connected to the blood-brain barrier by the circulatory system.

- The blood-brain barrier is to the brain what the mucosal gut barrier is to the gut. It acts as a second line of defense to protect the delicate central nervous system from dangerous toxins and organisms.

- The healthy bacteria of the gut produce molecules that maintain a tight blood-brain barrier. If the gut is unhealthy, the blood-brain barrier becomes loose and unhealthy.

- The healthy bacteria of the gut produce many of the same neurotransmitters as the brain and can use them to communicate with the brain.

CHAPTER 9:

HORMONES

To BE OR NOT TO be. That's the hormonal question. To be happy or sad, to be calm or aggressive, to be energetic or fatigued, involved or withdrawn, hungry or satisfied, alert or disinterested, hot or cold. In many ways, it does seem logical to blame our behavior on our hormones.

Hormones are complex. They are enveloped by a great deal of mystery and it certainly requires a great deal of skill to interpret and manipulate them. They interact in a delicate balance that seems almost impossible to harmonize and maintain. It reminds me of a beautiful spider's web. Once completed, the intricacy and beauty is astounding, but how easily it is dismantled!

In my own life, hormones have seemed to be my mortal enemies more than my intimate friends. My medical records are littered with hormones gone amuck and exasperating attempts to rebuild that delicate web. Throughout my 20s and into my 30s, I vainly hoped to restore my emotional and menstrual normalcy with bioidentical progesterone cream. A compounded thyroid medication was supposed to pull me out of my heavy cloud of fatigue and impart an intense desire to conquer the world. Then there were the adrenal supportive herbs that claimed to bring resiliency and give me a suit of armor against the emotional and physical threats that rained down upon me. Finally, I threw up my hands in surrender to the will of my hormones, striking a truce and allowing them to do as they pleased, learning to listen to them instead. Interestingly, it was then that I began to find respite from the turmoil.

Small yet mighty, hormones drive some of the most important activities of life. Hormones are composed of chains of amino acids, uniquely folded into specific shapes that determine their function. They are produced by glands in the body, which are part of the endocrine system. The gut is considered one of the largest endocrine glands in the body because it produces more than 100 molecules with hormonal action.[55]

Hormones are divided into classes that target specific organs. Together, they maintain our growth, metabolism, reproduction, mood, emotions, sleep, wakefulness, and last but not least, our stress response.

Let's consider some of the body's primary endocrine organs and the hormones they produce.

PITUITARY GLAND

- Adrenocorticotrophic hormone (ACTH): stimulates the adrenal gland
- Human growth hormone (HGH): promotes tissue and cell growth
- Thyroid-stimulating hormone (TSH): stimulates the thyroid gland
- Follicle-stimulating hormone (FSH): reproduction
- Prolactin: milk production
- Luteinizing hormone (LH): stimulates estrogen, progesterone, testosterone
- Antidiuretic hormone (ADH): increases water retention
- Oxytocin: milk production

HYPOTHALAMUS

- Thyrotropin-releasing hormone: stimulates TSH and prolactin
- Corticotropin-releasing hormone: triggers release of ACTH
- Gonadotropin-releasing hormone: triggers release of FSH and LH
- Growth hormone-releasing hormone: triggers release of HGH

ADRENAL GLAND

- Cortisol: stress response
- Estrogen: reproduction
- Testosterone: reproduction
- Adrenaline (epinephrine): stimulates nervous system
- Noradrenaline (norepinephrine): stimulates nervous system
- Dehydroepiandrosterone (DHEA): precursor to sex hormones
- Aldosterone: balances electrolytes

THYROID GLAND

- Thyroxine (T4): energy production
- Triiodothyronine (T3): energy production
- Calcitonin: regulates calcium

PARATHYROID GLAND

- Parathyroid hormone: regulates calcium

GONADS (OVARIES OR TESTES)

- Testosterone: reproduction
- Estrogen: reproduction
- Progesterone: reproduction, influences mood

PINEAL GLAND

- Melatonin: induces sleep, influences mood

PANCREAS

- Insulin: decreases blood sugar
- Glucagon: increases blood sugar

GUT

- Ghrelin: stimulates appetite
- Leptin: controls appetite
- Secretin: stimulates enzyme production

HYPOTHALAMUS-PITUITARY-ADRENAL AXIS (HPA AXIS)

The HPA axis is a unique subset of the endocrine system that represents the interactions of three glands: the hypothalamus, pituitary, and adrenal glands. Together, these glands regulate our body's response to stress.

Imagine you are driving down the road and an oncoming car begins to move into your lane. Your heart rate increases, your breathing accelerates, and you feel a surge of adrenaline that causes you to limit your focus to the immediate danger. This lifesaving response is the "adrenaline rush" that controls our reactions to perceived threats. The HPA axis controls this response.

In a nutshell, when the neurological system perceives a threat, it gives a direct command to headquarters (the hypothalamus), which releases an order in the form of corticotropin-releasing hormone. This order is immediately delivered to the commander (the pituitary gland), which establishes the directives (ACTH) for the officer (the adrenal gland). The officer then gives the order to fire the chemical agent, cortisol, into the body.

IMBALANCED HORMONES

The chronic stress we allow into our lives creates serious problems for our endocrine glands as they become overtaxed by constant demands. Jobs with urgent deadlines, hectic family schedules, traffic jams, constant electronic notifications, and continual waves of information overload our lives, leaving us little time for rest, relaxation, and deeply satisfying relationships. We are choosing to live lifestyles that place high demands on our HPA axis and threaten our delicate web of hormones.

Let's consider the following web of hormones:

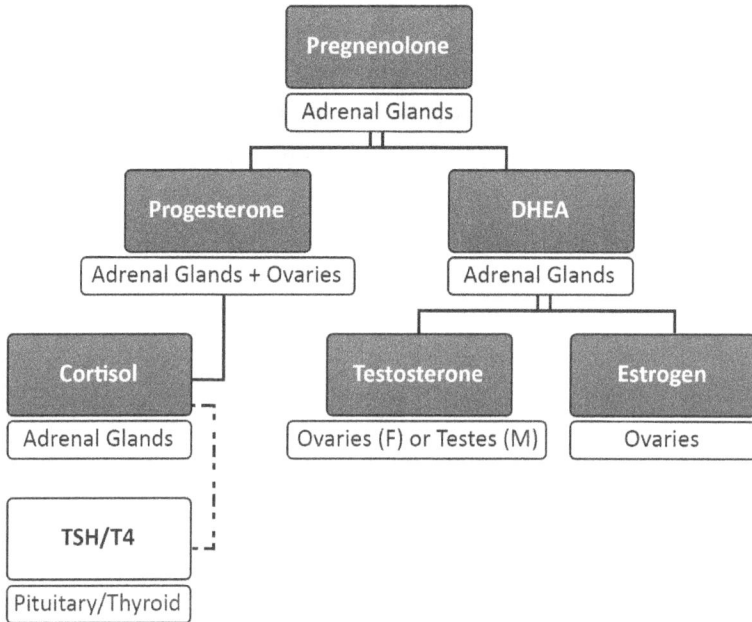

As the HPA axis operates in high gear, pregnenolone directs all resources toward the cortisol pathway, leaving other pathways deficient. DHEA, estrogen, and testosterone production slows. Even progesterone becomes scarce as the resources push more and more toward cortisol production. As you can see, the constant need for cortisol creates some significant deficiencies in sex hormones.

Cortisol communicates with other hormone pathways, such as the thyroid hormones. It inhibits the production of TSH and T4, leading to a temporary state of hypothyroidism. The primary indication of hypothyroidism is crippling fatigue.

Many of my own physical challenges were rooted in years of unhealthy habits, stressful circumstances, and an uncertain future. While completing my graduate degree, working various jobs, and attempting to maintain family responsibilities, I became increasingly plagued by various symptoms. I knew my energy was dwindling but dismissed it, convincing myself the situation was temporary. Late nights—or should I say, early mornings—left me frequently sick and drained of energy. Finally, I visited my functional medicine physician, hoping for an easy fix, but instead discovered I had a long battle ahead.

Amid this stress, my family sold our peaceful country home and prepared to move out of state. During this time, we moved to five homes within four years, including an inner-city home situated next to the residence of a busy drug dealer. The frequent late-night parties, fights, and police visits at our neighbor's house increased my stress further.

It was also during this time that several family members were diagnosed with chronic Lyme disease. We searched for answers and health practitioners we could trust while attempting various treatment regimens that were costly and tedious to manage. After making our final move, we found ourselves in unfamiliar territory with very few relationships or support systems.

These stressful years took a toll on my body. My adrenal glands struggled and began to assume control over the hormone cascade, stealing resources from other hormone pathways to maintain adequate amounts of cortisol. In this process, excess cortisol began to inhibit the production of my thyroid hormones, leaving me feeling like a wrung-out rag. Although I could sleep for 10 hours each night, I still woke up exhausted and needed naps to get through my day.

To make matters worse, as cortisol was stealing all the resources from my hormonal pathways, my estrogen and progesterone dropped significantly, making my menstrual cycles and moods unmanageable.

HORMONES AND THE GUT

So what does any of this have to do with the gut? Everything!

All hormones are interwoven into a tight complex that affects the gut. Therefore, one of the most common (but least recognized) symptoms of imbalanced hormones is gut distress. An overtaxed HPA axis creates an increasingly unhealthy gut, evidenced by bloating, pain, dysbiosis, and leaky gut. Much like the gut-brain axis, a two-way street runs between the gut and the HPA axis so that either system can affect the other.

Cortisol interacts with the gut as it:

- depresses the immune system and decreases the production of sIgA
- increases the body's need for glucose (energy), causing intense carb cravings and unstable blood sugar levels
- makes cells resistant to insulin, increasing carb cravings and causing weight gain
- induces the body's inflammatory response

All these events dismantle the mucosal gut barrier, increasing the risk of infections and leading to a variety of digestive problems. I also became the victim of cortisol-induced gut damage. The piercing abdominal pain, constant bloating, stomach ulcer, and increasing food intolerances finally led me to seek help for my chaotic hormones.

Cortisol can negatively affect the health of the gut over time, but our gut health also impacts our response to stress. An unhealthy gut exacerbates the response of the HPA axis because dysbiosis and leaky gut are additional stressors on the body. Harmful bacteria, yeast, and parasites dispatch communications through the vagus nerve, alerting the brain to their presence and serving as one more stressor on the HPA axis.[56]

On the other hand, a healthy gut with plenty of good bacteria can help the HPA axis deal with stressors. As the bacteria assist the immune system in fighting off physical threats in the gut, the enteric nervous system lets the brain know help is at hand and the HPA axis is disengaged from this battle.[57] Instead, it can focus its attention on more important stressors.

An overactive HPA axis can be the largest obstacle to healing, because it creates hormonal chaos and destroys the gut. Stress management is a critical requirement for good health.

In the next chapter, we will explore several ways that you can manage chronic stress in your life. Removing the stressor of an unhealthy gut is one way we can support our HPA axis.

THE PROBLEM: HASHIMOTO'S THYROIDITIS

Hashimoto's, the cause of nearly 90 percent of all hypothyroid conditions, is an autoimmune condition linked to the gut. In this condition, the body's immune system decides the thyroid gland is an enemy. It begins to attack the cells of this endocrine gland, leaving them beaten, bruised, and unable to function.

In a previous chapter, we learned how dysbiosis could be the root of autoimmunity issues. Untreated dysbiosis is unrelenting as it forces the immune system into a long battle. Eventually, exhaustion and weakened reserves cause the immune system to become sloppy in its surveillance of friend and foe.

Hashimoto's thyroiditis is one of many autoimmune conditions assumed to be triggered by a viral or allergenic threat in the gut. The invading virus or allergen contains proteins that are structurally similar to cells in the thyroid gland. As the overwhelmed immune system attempts to identify the intruder, it mistakenly marks the thyroid cells as foreign, leading to autoimmunity reactions.[58]

Research supports the connection between dysbiosis and autoimmune forms of hypothyroidism. There is evidence of unique types of bacteria found in the gut of those with hypothyroidism, indicating a relationship between gut microbiota and thyroid function.[59]

THE PROBLEM: POLYCYSTIC OVARY SYNDROME (PCOS)

Polycystic ovary syndrome (PCOS) is among the most frequently encountered gynecological issues in women of reproductive age. This condition represents yet another health challenge associated with poor gut health.

PCOS is an endocrine condition characterized by elevated male hormones (testosterone), disrupted menstruation, and metabolic complications such as cardiovascular risk factors, diabetes and blood sugar problems, and obesity. PCOS is an underlying cause for anovulation (inability to ovulate) and infertility.

A high-sugar, high-fat diet that fosters dysbiosis and leaky gut is a primary trigger of PCOS. This diet activates the immune system and encourages it to interfere with insulin receptors on the cells. The cells are unable to absorb sugar appropriately, forcing it to remain in the blood and leading to the high blood sugar characteristic of PCOS. The pancreas attempts to produce more insulin to lower the blood sugar, but it is unsuccessful, since the cells will not cooperate. High levels of insulin boost the production of testosterone, leading to PCOS.

When we correct dysbiosis, it calms the immune system so the cells begin responding to insulin and the production of excess testosterone ceases. Studies validate this idea by examining a distinct change in gut microbiota in individuals with PCOS following treatment for dysbiosis. The cells became more responsive to insulin, lowering the blood sugar and resolving many symptoms of PCOS.[60]

THE PROBLEM: OBESITY

Obesity is clearly one of the most important global challenges of our day, and an unhealthy gut is one cause. You may be wondering why I am addressing obesity in a chapter on hormones. I assure you, it is not a mistake. Hormones produced by the gut and pancreas such as insulin, ghrelin, and leptin regulate our appetites and how our body uses energy from the food we eat. Many other hormone-related conditions such as PCOS and diabetes are linked to obesity, too.

The rising obesity epidemic has spearheaded fervent research on this topic, and many studies point to the gut microbiota. The composition and quantity of the gut microbiota in obese individuals is very different from that of healthy individuals. The types of bacteria found in obese individuals are more efficient at extracting calories from the food. For example, the microbiota in obese individuals can break down indigestible fibers and turn them into glucose (sugar). This glucose becomes extra calories. In individuals with a healthy gut microbiota, the indigestible fibers would pass through the intestine and get eliminated. Therefore, the gut microbiota of obese individuals may be causing them to absorb more calories from their food.

The gut microbiota of obese individuals can also turn on genes that affect the way the body metabolizes carbohydrates and fats, causing them to be stored rather than used for energy.[61] Finally, the bacteria send messages to the brain through the vagus nerve that increase appetite and decrease satiety. As the bacteria affect eating behavior, they cause weight gain by increasing the appetite and decreasing the feeling of satiety.[62]

Many obese individuals consume a high-sugar, high-carbohydrate, processed diet with very few fresh, natural foods. This type of diet feeds yeast and bacteria, leading to dysbiosis and SIBO. The altered gut microbiota creates cravings for unhealthy foods that promote obesity.

THE PROBLEM: DIABETES

Type 1 diabetes is an autoimmune disease. Historically, type 2 diabetes has been the result of poor diet and lifestyle choices. For this reason, it has been coined "adult-onset" diabetes because it most often occurs in adults. Sadly, the tide is turning and we are witnessing children with this condition. Could this be a result of poor diet and inactivity? Or could this be a result of harmful microbiota passed on to children from mothers whose guts were unhealthy? Most likely, it is a combination of both. The research is clear, though: individuals with type 2 diabetes possess harmful gut microbiota, but when corrected, their diabetes improves.

A disrupted insulin system defines all forms of diabetes. Type 1 diabetes is marked by autoimmune reactions against the insulin-producing cells of the pancreas. Once the immune system destroys all these cells, insulin isn't produced to assist in sugar absorption. Therefore, sugar accumulates in the blood, reaching dangerously high levels.

Type 2 diabetes is not an autoimmune condition. Instead, the cells of the body no longer respond to insulin's prompts to "open up" and absorb sugar in the blood. This phenomenon is called insulin resistance. The pancreas secretes more insulin in response to the high blood sugar, but as the cells resist the insulin, the blood sugar continues to escalate. High-sugar, high-carbohydrate diets that require the continuous production of insulin may exhaust the cells' sensitivity to this hormone, rendering them resistant. A lack of activity spurs this resistance, since physical activity forces cells to accept glucose.

If you identify insulin resistance early, changes in dietary and lifestyle choices are often sufficient to persuade the cells to rethink their attitude toward insulin. If insulin resistance persists, the pancreas no longer produces insulin and you have a situation very similar to type 1 diabetes.

Obesity often precedes type 2 diabetes, and the trajectory of these conditions is similar. They also share a similar composition of gut bacteria. The microbiota of a healthy gut can favorably turn excess food energy (calories) into metabolic energy, which supports weight loss and decreases the risk of diabetes.

High blood sugar generates systemic inflammation, which is responsible for causing the long-term consequences of diabetes. A healthy gut microbiota can mitigate systemic inflammation and improve the trajectory of diabetes. As with obesity, a high-sugar, high-carbohydrate diet alters the microbiota to favor the development of type 2 diabetes. The unhealthy gut is both a result of and an exacerbating factor in the development and management of type 2 diabetes.

Chapter Summary: The gut microbiota maintains close connections with some of our core hormonal pathways and can influence them favorably or unfavorably. Hormones involved in the stress response, thyroid function, reproduction, and energy metabolism are affected by dysbiosis, immune activation, and inflammation. Therefore, we can conclude that hormonal imbalances are yet another group of health conditions rooted in the gut.

Key Points

- Hormones are chemicals that communicate with specific tissues, producing a particular action. Hormones regulate our growth, metabolism, reproduction, mood and emotion, sleep, and stress response.

- The HPA axis (including the hypothalamus, pituitary, and adrenal glands) is responsible for regulating our body's response to stress.

- When the body is under stress, the HPA axis releases the hormone cortisol.

- Chronic stress is marked by a continual demand for cortisol, which can lead to imbalanced hormones.

- Sustained high levels of cortisol depress the immune system, promote gut infections and inflammation, and destroy the mucosal gut barrier.

- Stress is one of the main causes of dysbiosis and leaky gut.

- Dysbiosis and chronic inflammation weaken the immune system; it becomes "lazy" and mistakes normal tissues as foreign. This process is called an autoimmune response and may be the underlying cause for many autoimmune conditions.

- Dysbiosis and problems metabolizing sugar can also affect sex hormones such as testosterone, causing imbalances and leading to conditions such as PCOS.

- Specific forms of bacteria in the gut can activate genes that promote obesity and send incorrect messages to the brain regarding appetite and feelings of satiety, contributing to weight gain and diabetes.

CHAPTER 10:

STRESS

A s I sat in the office of my naturopathic physician, listening to him rattle off the results of my most recent hormone and metabolic tests, I was shocked and confused. I could no longer hide behind the façade of a confident disposition that radiated a false message that everything was fine. Nope. The lab results laid bare my reality. They told of the internal race, the mental and physical fight, the exhaustion, and the depression. And they explained why bloating, abdominal pain, and gut distress had been my constant companions despite my fastidious diet, along with all the herbs, enzymes, and probiotics.

I tried to keep listening to the deep, methodical voice of my physician as he proceeded to tell me he had rarely seen a cortisol level as high as mine and that I was physiologically similar to a patient on prednisone. In addition to his previous suggestions of various adaptogenic herbs and lifestyle changes to reduce stress, his next recommendation hit me like a flash of lightning. Cognitive behavioral therapy. What? Now I wanted to fight rather than cry. I wasn't in need of counseling and brain therapy! If my cortisol had been high when I urinated on those test strips in the comfort of my home, I'm sure it jumped up several notches as I sat in the chair, thoughts reeling.

As I drove home, tears streamed down my face. I was discouraged, but knew I had to fight my enemy before it won the battle over my health. At least my enemy was now clearly identified: stress.

Stress is quickly becoming a modern-day epidemic. Even Merriam-Webster defines stress as "a physical, chemical, or emotional factor that causes bodily or mental tension and may be a factor in disease causation."[63] Yet stress itself is not the real problem: the body's response to it is. The adrenal glands are our body's tension indicators, and once stress is detected, a cascade of events occurs that includes the secretion and circulation of cortisol, the stress hormone.

Cortisol wreaks havoc on your entire body. It triggers systemic inflammation and destroys the gut. The fight-and-flight response generated by cortisol should rescue you from immediate danger or get you through a temporary crisis, but it was never designed to command your entire body indefinitely. And yet it does, and becomes the most destructive enemy we face. For those who have worked hard to choose a healthy lifestyle, eat a clean diet, drink purified water, and cleanse their environment, cortisol can shatter years of hard work. If you feel like you have labored to gain good health but are still fighting to keep your head above water, stress may be your root problem. If any of us expect to achieve and maintain an authentic state of health and vitality, stress management is not optional. It is required.

In this chapter, I want to share 20 ways to cultivate rest and calm in your life. These will help you reduce stress, lower cortisol, and support your body's natural ability to heal itself. Think of stress management as cleaning your home. If you neglect to clean, the chaos and filth become overwhelming. It is much easier to maintain a clean home than to remove years of dirt and clutter. Practicing daily stress management keeps your body cleansed of excess cortisol and makes it simpler and even pleasant for the body to do its normal jobs.

In some ways, this chapter concludes the narrative on *why* healing the gut is important for establishing a healthy life. But it also introduces our next narrative on *how* to heal the gut. Stress management is foundational for healing anything, including the gut. It creates the environment in which all other healing modalities can perform effectively. Without stress management, you may experience some improvements in your health, but you will not experience your body's full health potential. Symptoms will linger and healing will seem just barely out of reach. As you proceed through this chapter, consider lifestyle changes you can make to reduce your stress and prepare your body for the specific dietary changes we will discuss next.

20 WAYS TO CULTIVATE CALM

Cultivate a Calm Body

1. **Breathe Deeply**. Most of us take short, shallow breaths. Take the time to observe yourself breathing. Do your shoulders and chest rise, or does your belly expand and fall back? Deep breathing comes from the belly and is, logically, called belly breathing. Infants naturally breathe from their belly. Stress causes us to take short, shallow breaths that don't adequately oxygenate our tissues or brain. Deep belly breathing tells our body to calm down and relax. Have you ever noticed yourself intuitively heaving a deep sigh when you are stressed? It's your body's way of forcing you to breathe deeply and relax.

    Stress increases your heart and respiratory rates, but deep breathing reduces them. Those who practice deep breathing can calm a nervous system that is activated by stress. Deep breathing also enhances the immune system and oxygenates the brain so you can mentally and physically manage stress.

2. **Sleep at the Right Time**. When we are under stress, sleep eludes us. We become wired in the evening, have trouble falling asleep, or cannot stay asleep. Out of frustration, this often leads to poor sleep habits in which we stay up late or sleep in. Not only does stress cause disordered sleep, but poor sleep schedules can cause chronic stress. Busy schedules that force us to become night owls weaken our defenses and trigger the stress response. Adrenal fatigue[g] is one of the most common examples of this scenario.

    The body's restoration phase cycles with our circadian rhythm. All our body's organ systems, and especially the adrenal glands, perform the greatest amount of repairs between the hours of 10 p.m. and 2 a.m. If we are not sleeping during that time, we are robbing our body

---

g   A condition in which chronic stress exhausts the adrenal glands, leading to fatigue, insomnia, pain, and changes in hormones and neurotransmitters.

of its ability to prepare for the next day. Have you ever noticed that routine late nights or working third shift makes you more susceptible to getting sick? This phenomenon occurs because the immune system is not being adequately restored at night and becomes weak.

The adrenal glands must be functioning at peak performance to manage stress appropriately. Therefore, sleeping between 10 p.m. and 2 a.m. is one of the best ways to increase your stamina and fight stress.

3. **Take Epsom Salt Baths**. Soaking in a tub of warm water with at least two cups of Epsom salts calms the mind and relaxes the body. Epsom salts contain magnesium, a mineral that relaxes tight muscles. Most of us are severely magnesium deficient because stress depletes our body of this calming mineral. Magnesium decreases inflammation, and especially inflammation of the neurological system. It has been shown to promote better mood and sleep because of its positive effects on the brain. Magnesium is not absorbed well in the gut but readily passes through the skin, making an Epsom salt bath an ideal way to replenish this mineral.

4. **Generate Endorphins through Light Exercise**. Endorphins are neurotransmitters that promote good feelings. They reduce our perception of pain, similar to opiates, and decrease feelings of stress. Light exercises such as stretching, walking, yoga, and swimming generate endorphins. Intense activity also produces endorphins, but it produces cortisol as well, making it a poor choice for stress management. Optimal forms of exercise vary for everyone. Some people require more intense activity to generate endorphins, while very little activity is sufficient for others. Taking walks is an excellent way to pump some "happy" chemicals into your nervous system and reduce stress.

5. **Develop a Morning and Bedtime Routine**. Life can get crazy, but establishing and maintaining a morning and bedtime routine will do wonders for managing stress. I have always enjoyed living spontaneously and fought routine, but this lack of self-discipline caused my health to fail on numerous occasions. After visiting my

naturopathic physician, I implemented my own behavioral changes. A large part of my healing became my established morning and bedtime routine. It changed my health and my life substantially.

My bedtime routine begins at 9 p.m. when all electronics are turned off or put on airplane mode to reduce blue light and electromagnetic radiation. Both components prevent the body from making melatonin, the hormone that helps you sleep. Despite having blue light filters on all my electronics, the electromagnetic radiation can still disrupt the natural circadian rhythm that promotes sleep. Therefore, reading on a tablet at night is not a good idea. Three nights each week, I take an Epsom salt bath for 20 to 30 minutes, with added calming essential oils, and practice deep breathing during the soak. By 10 p.m., I'm in bed, reading something encouraging, and aiming for lights out by 10:30.

Each morning at 6:30 a.m., my phone alarm begins its unobtrusive reminder that it is time to get out of bed. Yes, I use my phone as an alarm clock, but remember, it was put on airplane mode the night before to cancel the electromagnetic radiation. Please don't sleep with a cell phone by your bed unless it is in airplane mode. This practice has been linked to severe health consequences, especially in children.

As soon as I awake, I spend an hour reading my Bible to calm my mind, empty it of its worries and concerns, and gain a positive perspective for the day ahead. This practice is one form of mindful meditation, which is quickly developing into an essential element of health and wellness advocated by all health practitioners, traditional or holistic. Finally, my morning routine ends with 30 minutes of exercise before hopping into the shower and beginning my day.

After about three months of faithfully submitting to this routine, my energy improved, my outlook on life was more positive, and my resilience had increased. The stressors in my life had not changed, but my response to them did. This is how stress management can help you heal. As you can see, cultivating all five elements of a calm body isn't difficult, but it does take practice. Practice creates habits, and healing habits create health.

Cultivate a Calm Environment

6. **Avoid Sensory Overload**. Far too many of us live or work in an environment that blasts us with stimulation. Televisions, computer pop-ups, lights, and billboards inundate our visual fields. Likewise, our ears are bombarded with sounds of loud music, telephones, notifications, sirens, and conversations. Urban environments assault our noses with exhaust, cleaning chemicals, perfumes, and outgassing building materials. Our brain must interpret and respond to all these sensory inputs. Each of them is a potential stressor that increases our total stress load and distracts the body from healing. Compare our industrialized, digital world with the environment in which we were designed to reside. Nature offers us peaceful images without flashing advertisements, quiet sounds, and the healing aromas of natural essential oils. If we want our body to heal, we must be more conscious about reducing the sensory input that increases our stress response. Many of us have become apathetic about the stimulatory inputs surrounding us, but our bodies are not unaffected. Take inventory of the sensory input in your environment. If possible, turn off the television and the radio, and stop staring at the screens around you. We can't control all our environments, but those you *can* control can be places of rest rather than places of chaos.

7. **Stop Overcommitting**. Society has misled us to believe we must take every opportunity presented to us if we are to be well-rounded, successful individuals. This pressure is especially intense among school-aged children who are home only to sleep, otherwise being continually transported from one activity to another in the name of opportunity and personal development. But even adults are pressured into playing the roles of professional, parent, volunteer, and scholar simultaneously. Unfortunately, this lie—that we must do everything, all the time—has placed undue stress on children and adults alike. As the years pass, the pressures of commitments, social schedules, and personal advancement opportunities burden our bodies and rob us of time with ourselves, our families, our close friends, and those we could serve.

    Saying "no" to opportunities will not hold you back from success.

Rather, it fosters personal health and a value system that is far more advantageous to you overall. In previous centuries, sick individuals spent a significant amount of time in convalescence before resuming their normal lives. This time allowed freedom from commitments and responsibilities while enabling the body to heal. Today, we go to the doctor's office and grab a pill to ensure we can resume our normal activities without missing a beat. To achieve and maintain health, we must have periods of convalescence, and stop allowing the stress of overcommitment to control our lives.

8. **Minimize Clutter and Possessions**. Stuff requires our attention. After living in five homes over four years, my family rapidly learned the value of decluttering and getting rid of things. Stuff takes up space, time, and energy. Society would have us believe that our stuff is important and part of our identity—but the truth is, it devalues us as humans. Value lies in people, not things. Clutter and possessions take our time and resources, which increases our stress load. Minimize the stuff in your life, and your body will enjoy freedom from this pressure.

9. **Reduce Your Workload**. Workaholics are among the most unhealthy individuals. Statistically, they have shorter lifespans and are more likely to die suddenly. They push themselves to the brink and ignore all the warning signs of declining health until their bodies fail. The pressure to climb the corporate ladder to be financially successful robs us of the most valuable elements of life, such as relationships and health. Ironically, the wealthiest individuals often become the most unhappy when they realize money and professional status do not bring satisfaction. Workaholics maintain the highest levels of stress, and healing is nearly impossible under the weight of this burden.

10. **Take Time to Enjoy Nature**. Nature has the innate ability to reduce our burden of stress. It offers a serene environment that woos us into a state of reflection and peace. Taking hikes through the woods, sitting by water, climbing mountains, watching a sunrise or sunset, and even just playing in your own backyard allows you to breathe fresh air and take a break from the loud noises and visual stimulation of society. The sounds of nature reduce cortisol, even when you're

simply listening to recorded natural sounds. Engaging in light exercise while enjoying nature increases endorphins, which reduce pain and promote positive feelings. The essential oils released by plants offer healing aromatherapy. If you can enjoy nature "off the grid," your body will enjoy a reprieve from the electromagnetic radiation of cell phones, wireless networks, Bluetooth, and other destructive electronic networks.

11. **Aromatherapy**. Many essential oils reduce cortisol levels, lower your heart and breathing rates, and change neurotransmitters to diminish anxiety, depression, and stress. Lavender, rose, lemon balm, ylang-ylang, bergamot, chamomile, and frankincense are commonly used in diffusers or added to bathwater for their stress-reducing effects. Adding a diffuser to your work or home setting can help promote a calmer environment.

12. **Minimize Screen Time**. I believe we will soon learn of the detrimental effects of screens on our health, and especially that of our children. With the explosion of the digital age, our fascination with technology overrides good judgment. Within one generation, millions of people have become continually connected to electromagnetic devices as they carry cell phones on their body, work on computers and tablets for extended hours each day, and wear technology-based watches and wristbands. Is it even possible to live without technology? This generation of children is the first to be exposed to large amounts of electronic radiation from cell phones, computers, and tablets from conception.

The popular journal *Psychology Today* has cited several studies showing that screen time induced the physiological effects of stress (e.g., increased heart rate, breathing rate, cortisol levels), impaired digestion, and changed neurotransmitters to affect attention and sleep habits.[64] The blue light emitted from electronic screens is proven to cause sleep, hormone, and cognitive problems because it affects melatonin, an important hormone in the body.

Although we may think it is relaxing to sit down and watch television or a movie, the truth is that electronic screens induce stress and hinder healing.

13. **Music Therapy**. Music is a powerful medium with the ability to change our thoughts, emotions, and actions. Everywhere we go, music engulfs us, yet the choice of style is rarely therapeutic. Music was first introduced into stores because it caused shoppers to linger and purchase more. However, the classical "elevator" music found to produce those results has been replaced with the obnoxious music of pop culture, which is shown to promote aggression and irritation. The style of music played in public venues is no longer chosen based on desired outcomes but celebrity trends.

    Studies show nature's music produces the greatest reductions in cortisol, but calming music such as classical, spa, soft instrumental, and Celtic music also reduces anxiety, anger, and stress. Heavy metal, rap, hip-hop, and similar genres have been shown to increase irritability, anger, and cortisol, and can be a stressor. Unfortunately, much of the music that surrounds us does not promote relaxation, but contributes to the overload of stressful sensory input. Creating a relaxing environment with calming music helps reduce stress.

Cultivate a Calm Mind

14. **Pray and Meditate**. Prayer and meditation have significant effects on our stress response. Medical literature abounds with studies showing that those who have a strong faith system and an active religious belief are far happier and less stressed than those who do not. Faith, prayer, and meditation bring meaning, purpose, and perspective to life, allowing us to cultivate a renewed sense of hope. Personally, I can attest to the fact that all my efforts at reducing mental and emotional stress pale in comparison to the relief and peace I find when I surrender everything to my Lord and Savior, Jesus Christ. Knowing that I belong to One who governs the affairs of my life and communing with Him daily brings peace that extends beyond my understanding or ability to deliver to myself. We all have an innate need to worship, and prayer and meditation are how we worship.

15. **Be Grateful**. Gratitude is a powerful attitude that helps us to recognize and meditate on the positive things in life, rather than the negative. Negative experiences, situations, and relationships inherently cause physical, emotional, and mental stress. The more we ruminate upon

these negative experiences, the higher our cortisol levels grow and the greater burden of stress we place upon ourselves. We may not be able to run from negative experiences, but when we choose to consciously focus on the positive experiences and relationships we are grateful for, we can neutralize the negative experiences. The more gratitude you can express, the less mental and emotional stress you will experience.

16. **Give Generously**. Giving is a contagious experience that ameliorates stress. Generosity does not have to be monetary. Giving your time and attention can be far more rewarding than monetary gifts. Generosity requires you to focus on someone other than yourself, and the mere act of turning your eyes away from self and toward other's needs lowers your cortisol significantly, as well as generating endorphins. Your life has more meaning and purpose when you give yourself to others in ways that benefit them and society. Volunteer work provides opportunities to give generously, but be sure you are not overcommitting yourself. Giving also requires you to seek out the needs of others to discover ways you could give. Giving is a powerful way to calm a stressful mind by turning it toward others.

17. **Focus on People, Not Things**. Generosity naturally points us toward people and away from things. It is an initial step in learning to focus on people. The more we can focus on people, the less we focus on attaining and maintaining things. If we found ourselves alone on an island, we would not need a beautiful house, a new car, a large bank account, or a list of our professional or academic achievements. We would need people. Turning our mind away from the things of this world and toward people changes our perspective, goals, and desires. We become less consumed with possessions and accomplishments and start seeing areas where we can serve and give generously. A mind that is focused on others and not on things is far less stressed and more peaceful than one focused on gaining and maintaining things.

18. **Build Relationships**. We can begin focusing on people in general, but each of us has a desire and need to form deep relationships. We need to know there is a core group of people who know, love, and care for us. Most often, these people are our own family members, but

they can span further to a select group of close friends. Don't neglect building relationships with those closest to you.

Relationships are about more than just dwelling with or providing for another person. A good relationship requires constant work and involvement from each party to develop, nurture, and deepen. Marriage doesn't automatically establish a relationship between two people. They must work to establish and keep it. A familial connection such as a parent to a child does not ensure a relationship. Far too often, busy schedules, overcommitment, workaholism, and a focus on things have robbed us of potential relationships. We might cohabitate, but we don't truly have relationships, leading to family discord, jealousy, unfaithfulness, rebellion, and stress. I have never met a person who regretted building a true relationship, but I have met many people who deeply regretted not spending more time and attention on fostering a relationship with a spouse, child, family member, or friend while they had the opportunity. Humans were created to be relational, which is why isolation has repeatedly been associated with stress, health problems, and even death.

19. **Laugh More**. Laughing is one of the best medicines for stress, which is why conference speakers attempt to add humor to release tension in their listeners. Laughter is used to break the ice and make people feel comfortable with their surroundings or situation. It puts their minds at ease. Laughing not only makes you feel good emotionally, but it also generates endorphins that ameliorate pain, reduce cortisol levels, relax muscles, enhance memory, and boost immune function. Laughter is an inexpensive way to support a healthy mental attitude and reduce stress.

20. **Keep a Journal**. Many people find journaling to be a very calming activity that effectively reduces mental stress. Writing down thoughts can be a way to eliminate them from your mind, especially if they are negative thoughts and emotions. Journaling can allow you to problem-solve.

I have found it helpful to keep a journal of encouraging quotes, meaningful Scripture verses, and prayers. When my mind begins racing, worrying, and growing fearful and stress starts to weigh me down, I look back at these encouraging words as reminders that I have braved the storms of the past and can continue to do so.

After several months of implementing many of these new habits into my own life to cultivate calm and reduce stress, my health made a complete 180-degree turn. My energy levels were higher than they had been in years, my outlook on life was hopeful, my hormones began stabilizing, and my gut was finally starting to settle down. Stress affects us profoundly. Even today, when I fail to manage stress in my life, my health quickly begins to suffer, beginning with my gut.

I want to offer hope to those who may find themselves in stressful circumstances or relationships they can't change. I understand. We all have situations and circumstances that create ongoing stress. It is part of being human. The day stress disappears will be the day we are perfect people with perfect jobs, perfect families, perfect diets, perfect environments, and perfect thoughts. The reality is, we are fallen people living in a fallen world, but we have the resources to rise above our circumstances and situations and to live peaceful lives.

Corrie ten Boom helped many Jews escape the Nazi Holocaust of World War II before being imprisoned herself. She survived 10 months in one of the most horrendous German concentration camps and lost her entire family before her release. Her story and wisdom survive today and provide an incredible example of one woman who maintained an inner state of peace despite unchangeable and deplorable circumstances. Don't get discouraged if you find yourself in a situation that seems hopeless. It is possible to gain a sense of peace and physical healing by managing mental and physical stress.

"Happiness isn't something that depends on our surroundings…
it's something we make inside ourselves."

~ *Corrie ten Boom, Holocaust survivor*

PART 2:

THE DETAILS OF THE PLAN
WHY IS THIS THE SOLUTION?

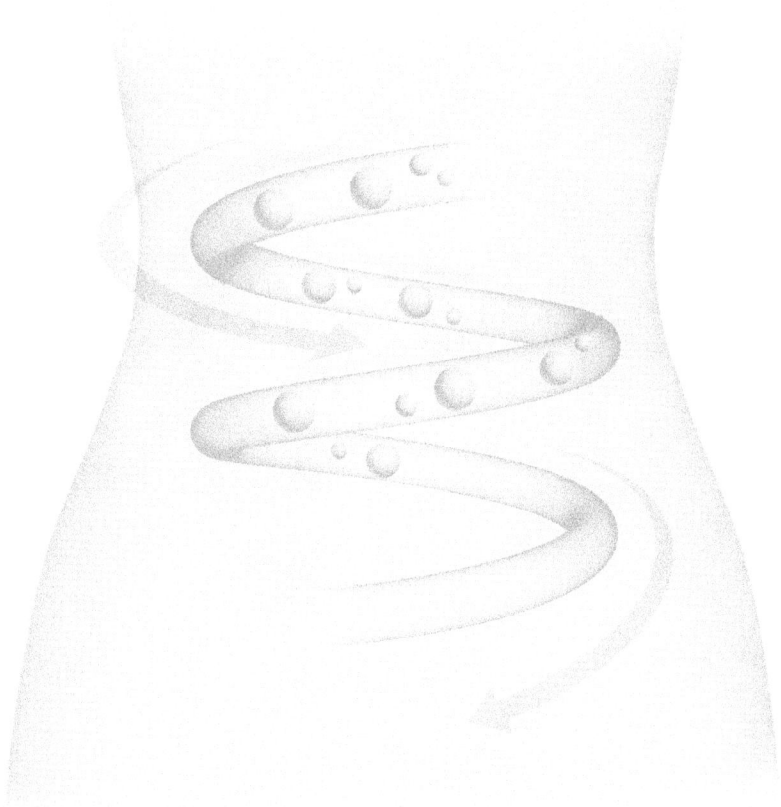

CHAPTER 11:

THE PLAN

"All disease begins in the gut."

~Hippocrates, 400 BC

DYSBIOSIS, LEAKY GUT, SIBO, INFLAMMATION, autoimmunity issues, childhood infections, *Candida*, parasites, stealth infections, toxicity, IBS/IBD, cardiovascular disease, cancer, autism, ADD/ADHD, dementia, depression, thyroiditis, PCOS, obesity, and diabetes—these health problems mark so many of our lives, or those of our loved ones.

Did Hippocrates, the father of modern medicine, hit the nail on the head centuries ago when he boldly concluded that all disease begins in the gut? And if he was correct, why is modern medicine just beginning to look at the gut and express surprise at its association with so many health conditions? Has it forgotten the truth revealed so long ago?

By now, I hope you have gained a better understanding of the connection between a healthy gut and a healthy life. There is hope for a new beginning if you have suffered long and painful battles with chronic illness. If you are willing to commit to a new lifestyle paradigm, you can begin to restore your health and experience vitality. In the following chapters, you will receive detailed instructions for putting your new plan into action.

Just what *is* this new plan, you ask? Let us again turn to ancient wisdom.

"Let food be thy medicine and medicine be thy food."

– Hippocrates, 400 BC

The gut is one of our most adaptable systems. It may break, but you can fix it. Sadly, human nature chooses to ignore or even accept the warning signals of a weak, struggling system. Oftentimes, we wait for a life-altering diagnosis before facing the seriousness of the threat. When the unavoidable condition becomes a reality, we then choose to begin the arduous task of repairing the broken system. The journey drives many to discover the benefits of maintaining a healthy life, which is far more appealing than accepting the temporary fixes offered by mainstream medicine.

As Hippocrates affirms, nutrition is an important part of the journey to a healthier life. A poor diet causes extensive damage to the gut, and we must restructure our diet if we hope to repair that broken system. Successfully fixing a gut that has been slowly falling apart over several years requires determination and commitment. We know a good maintenance plan is far less costly and time-consuming than the price we pay for years of neglect. Fortunately, the gut is a dynamic system, able to regenerate with proper nourishment and discipline.

Before we begin looking at the details of how to fix your gut, I want to encourage and redirect a special group of readers. If you have a history of an eating disorder, strong tendencies to eat emotionally, or a very challenging relationship with food, please find some help with these issues before embarking on the journey I lay out before you. This journey can be very difficult, as it involves temporarily eliminating some foods that people connect to emotionally. I don't want to see you get frustrated, feel like a failure, or sink deeper into emotional challenges. If you struggle with disordered or emotional eating, I highly suggest you read Heidi Schauster's book, *Nourish: How to Heal Your Relationship with Food, Body, and Self.* Heidi brings more than two decades of experience to the table and can help you reestablish a healthy relationship with food before you proceed through this plan.

THE "4R" PLAN

In the 1990s, Dr. Jeffrey Bland, PhD, of the Institute of Functional Medicine, created a program that systematically addressed all the necessary steps for healing the gut. The principles of this plan have been successfully implemented by many individuals to correct dysbiosis, SIBO, leaky gut, and systemic inflammation.

What is the "4R" Plan? From a bird's-eye view, the plan involves four steps, which the remainder of this chapter will dissect in greater detail.

1. **REMOVE:** Remove damaging foods, harmful microorganisms (bacteria, yeast, parasites), toxins, and stress, which all irritate the gut, make it leaky, and trigger immune reactions.

2. **REPAIR:** Repair the damaged villi, "leaky" cell junctions, and mucosal gut barrier with supportive foods and supplements.

3. **REPLACE**: Replace digestive enzymes to correct digestion while rebuilding villi.

4. **REINOCULATE**: Reinoculate the gut with healthy probiotics to rebalance the gut microbiota and restore the mucosal gut barrier.

The first step is the hardest to implement, but gives you the greatest leap toward healing. Most of us are stuck in habits of comfort and tend to be resistant to having our food choices redirected. Admittedly, the first step requires willpower and fortitude. You must learn to think differently about food and what you welcome into your body or home. Once you begin to associate your quality of health with your food choices, your new healthy choices become an attractive lifestyle instead of a forced diet plan. As your gut starts to heal, you will feel better, have more energy, and realize the amazing benefits of providing your body with nourishing foods. The next several chapters will educate you on the best food choices and nutraceuticals to help your gut heal and restore the foundation of your health.

The amount of time required to regenerate the gut is very personalized. If you are older and have eaten a poor diet since childhood, taken multiple antibiotics, and lived a stressful lifestyle, then you must stick with this plan for at least a year. If you don't have a history littered with perpetrators of poor gut health, six months may be sufficient to heal. In either case, this plan trains you to recognize and choose healthy eating patterns to maintain your gut health for years after finishing the "4R" plan.

Next, we will discuss the details of each of the four R's.

STEP 1: REMOVE

Healing begins when you eliminate the offenders that trigger dysbiosis, leaky gut, immune reactions, and inflammation. Removing these enemies is the hardest step of the plan since you are, quite literally, fighting a battle. Carefully selected foods and nutraceuticals are sent to help ambush the enemies. Despite its difficulty, removing the offenders in our gut is the most important step of healing because it allows the immune system to regroup, resupply, and focus attention on the wounded gut rather than the offenders.

The most notorious enemies to eliminate include:

- dangerous microorganisms (bacteria, yeast, and parasites),
- dietary allergens,
- inflammatory foods, and
- stress.

Let's look at how we will address each of these offenders.

Bacteria, Yeast, & Parasites

Dysbiosis or SIBO typically precedes a leaky gut, and as we discussed earlier in this book, good bacteria cannot grow when a large population of harmful bacteria, yeast, and parasites exists. The gut is similar to a community, and the families that settle there will populate the community with their friends and relatives. The host's defense weapons against unfriendly communities are specific foods (nourishment) and targeted nutraceuticals.

Nourishment (Food): Bacteria and yeast use the foods we consume to obtain energy and repopulate the gut. Fortunately, these microorganisms have selective eating habits. They prefer to feast on glucose (i.e., sugar), which is supplied by carbohydrates. These include sugar, grains, fruit, and starchy vegetables. The bacteria and yeast do not like non-starchy veggies because they provide few glucose molecules. Direct sources of sugar (white and brown sugar, honey, maple syrup, etc.) serve up a feast of glucose. As we will see in Chapter 12, it is necessary to eliminate most sweeteners, while Chapters 13 and 16 direct us to temporarily reduce most grains, fruits, and starchy vegetables in order to remove the food sources for bacteria, yeast, and parasites.

White, refined grain or flour also provides an abundance of glucose because it contains pure starch—large strands of bound glucose molecules. As digestive enzymes disassemble the starch, glucose is released and the microorganisms begin to feast. All white, refined grain must be eliminated from your diet to remove harmful organisms from the gut.

Fruit is a source of glucose, although it provides less than pure sugar or white, refined grains. High-sugar fruits, like bananas and dried fruit, supply the gut with more glucose than low-sugar fruits like grapefruit and berries. In Chapter 16, we will learn how to choose low-sugar fruits while healing the gut.

All grains, including whole grains, contain a lot of starch, which becomes glucose through the process of digestion. Whole grains release glucose at a much slower rate because a hard shell of bran encases the starch. Digestive enzymes must first remove the bran before accessing the starch. Therefore, whole grains don't feed microorganisms as quickly as refined grain. If you have an extremely unhealthy gut, it will be necessary to temporarily remove all grains from your diet because of their starch content, but others may be able to consume some forms of gluten-free, whole grains, as we will learn in Chapter 13.

High-starch vegetables such as potatoes also offer a quick source of glucose and supply bacteria and yeast with a nice meal, so they should be eliminated while we remove the harmful organisms. High-starch vegetables will be classified in Chapter 16.

Fat and protein are valuable nutrients for healing because they don't provide glucose for bacteria and yeast. The microorganisms starve when glucose is limited, and that is the result we're seeking. Therefore, fat and protein become important elements of a gut-healing diet.

The goal of the "4R" healing diet is to eliminate sources of food that nourish dangerous microorganisms in the gut. If we cut off their food supply, we can remove the harmful microorganisms through starvation. Chapters 12 through 20 will guide you through each food group and help you choose foods that heal the gut and learn which foods to eliminate because they feed dangerous microorganisms.

Nutraceuticals: To expedite the battle, we use antimicrobial herbal supplements to help kill harmful bacteria, yeast, and parasites. Some herbals target specific families of microorganisms, so it is important to use a combination of herbs for the best results. Bacteria and yeast also develop resistance toward antimicrobial agents (whether pharmaceutical or nutraceutical). For this reason, it is important to switch agents frequently to avoid this damaging behavior. Please consult with a functional medicine practitioner regarding specific dosages for each nutraceutical, as many individual factors may impact your specific dosing needs.

Some of the best antimicrobial herbals include the following:

For bacteria:

- Oregano oil
- Olive leaf extract
- Garlic (allicin)
- Grapefruit seed extract
- Berberines (a potent antimicrobial compound extracted from several herbs)
- Chinese skullcap
- Licorice root (*Glycyrrhiza glabra*)

For yeast:

- Garlic (allicin)
- Caprylic acid
- Berberines
- Grape seed extract (not to be confused with grapefruit seed extract)
- Oregano oil
- Cat's claw

For parasites:

- Goldenseal
- Artemisia (wormwood)
- Oregano oil
- Black walnut
- Grapefruit seed extract
- Garlic
- Clove
- Diatomaceous earth

Many families of bacteria and yeast create a sticky, mucus-like covering around their colony. This cover is called a biofilm, and it provides protection from antimicrobial agents. Biofilms are one cause of antibiotic resistance and have presented a dangerous situation for medicine. In well-established *Candida* infections or dysbiosis, specific enzymes are required to dissolve this biofilm, exposing the bacteria or yeast colony to further attack. We call these enzymes "biofilm busters." They ensure the antimicrobial herbals have access to the villains.

Effective biofilm busters include:

- Grapefruit seed extract
- Nattokinase
- Serrapeptase
- Thyme essential oil
- DNase
- Licorice root

Food Allergens & Inflammatory Foods

Food allergens trigger a destructive immune response and inflammation, as well as fueling leaky gut. Healing the gut requires the elimination of all actual food allergens. The difficulty lies in determining what foods are actual allergens. Dysbiosis and leaky gut can indicate false food allergens or sensitivities on a food allergy test. The labeled allergens may be false because these foods wouldn't be allergenic if the gut was healthy. A leaky gut causes undigested food particles to enter the bloodstream. The immune system identifies them as foreign invaders and responds like they are a food allergy. A healthy gut has tight junctions that keep undigested food particles out of the bloodstream, preventing an allergic response. Therefore, many alleged food allergies resolve after we heal the gut.

However, some foods cause true allergic reactions in a significant portion of the population. These include:

- gluten,
- dairy,
- peanuts,
- corn, and
- soy.

As a general rule, most of us should avoid these common food allergens while healing the gut. Other individual food allergens that you may have to avoid can only be determined through a high-quality food allergy test, which can be provided by a functional medicine practitioner.

We should also avoid foods that cause inflammation because the gut won't heal in an inflamed environment. These include food preservatives and additives, gluten, dairy, soy, corn, and all refined grains and oils. We will revisit these foods in future chapters. Each triggers the immune system to initiate inflammation and is a roadblock to healing.

A healing diet must include whole foods that are free from unnatural processing and ingredients such as preservatives, additives, pesticides, herbicides, and artificial colors and flavorings. Processed, unnatural foods aren't just inflammatory—they deliver toxins to the body and act as a stressor on our organ systems. An inflamed, toxic body won't heal.

Stress
The last enemy we must remove is stress. This enemy is, perhaps, the most difficult to deal with, as many of us live modern lifestyles that foster stress. As we strive to fulfill our dreams and ambitions, we incur the burden of more responsibility, more time constraints, less time for exercise or activity, and even less time for meal planning and preparation. We mark success by putting in long hours, ascending the corporate ladder, and gaining thriving careers. Sadly, health is not considered a mark of success today. In fact, our health is often the price we pay for corporate success. A sudden health crisis may temporarily slow us down, but we settle for a quick fix and return to our fast pace as soon as possible.

Dysfunctional or absent relationships also cause substantial stress. Superficiality and loneliness pervade our society as young and old alike fail to gain any real sense of purpose. Relationships, hope, and purpose are essential to our well-being. When these are lacking, the mental stress created soon affects our gut and health.

In the previous chapter, we learned the adrenal glands act as our body's stress response system. This system was intended to function in short-term situations, but becomes increasingly depleted as the duration of stress lengthens. The adrenal glands secrete an inflammatory hormone called cortisol into our bloodstream to alert other organ systems of the threat of stress. As cortisol levels rise, the mucus barrier and fragile villi of the gut become inflamed and weakened. Long-term stress, marked by excessive cortisol levels, eventually damages the villi, leading to leaky gut and systemic inflammation.

We must recognize stress as an enemy of healing we must remove. Review the 20 ways to cultivate calm in Chapter 10 if stress is a significant companion in your life.

STEP 2: REPAIR

After we remove the offenders attacking the gut, we can begin repairing the injured gut. This second step focuses on rebuilding the damaged villi, closing the tight junctions between the cells of the intestine, reconstructing the mucosal gut barrier, and restoring the immune system. This process takes the longest to accomplish. The longer a gut has been inflamed and leaky, the greater the destruction, creating the need for more substantial repair. A severely destroyed gut may take up to a year to fix. The cells of a younger person are more flexible and heal more quickly. Therefore, we can repair a child's gut much more quickly than an adult's gut.

Nutraceuticals aid in the repair process by managing inflammation and supplying nutrients required for rebuilding intestinal cells. The following nutraceuticals are essential for repair:

- **Omega-3 fatty acids**: These fatty acids are among the most potent anti-inflammatory agents and are used to manage various inflammatory conditions. They are a vital part of your daily health routine. Fish oil is the most common omega-3 fatty acid. Be careful, though: not all fish oils are created equal. It is important to choose a high-quality, purified fish oil free from contaminants (PCBs, cadmium, arsenic, lead, dioxins), and which is fresh. It must deliver adequate amounts of EPA and DHA (the key anti-inflammatory compounds) and must be sourced from wild-caught fish. Many commercial fish oils are rancid and contaminated, increasing the amount of damaging free radicals in the body, which is counterproductive to healing.

Recommendation: 1–2 grams of omega-3 fatty acids, taken daily.

- **Glutamine**: Also known as L-glutamine, this amino acid is a primary food source for the villi. It helps rebuild damaged villi and close the tight junctions that cause leaky gut. It maintains both the structure and integrity of the villi.

  Recommendation: 2–4 grams of glutamine, taken daily in divided doses.

- **Zinc**: This mineral has often been used to decrease "leakiness" in the gut of individuals with Crohn's disease and other conditions associated with increased gut permeability.[65] It helps to clear the mucosal gut barrier of infectious organisms, preventing them from damaging the intestinal walls. Zinc maintains an environment that favors healing, is critical for cell function, and helps the cells reform tight junctions.

  Recommendation: 30–60mg daily.

- **Vitamin D**: Research links many autoimmune and intestinal inflammatory conditions such as IBS and IBD to a vitamin D deficiency. This vital nutrient boosts the function of the immune system by activating the production and function of various immune cells. It supports both innate and adaptive immune responses and is a natural anti-inflammatory. For this reason, the media and researchers have given focused attention to the role of vitamin D in chronic health conditions. Vitamin D rebuilds the immune system and quenches inflammation, while other nutrients focus on the villi and mucosal gut barrier.

  Recommendation: 2,000IU of vitamin D daily. (Many individuals are deficient and initially need more. I suggest testing before supplementing.)

Advanced cases of SIBO, gastrointestinal distress, abdominal pain, and bloating require additional nutraceuticals that soothe and protect the damaged gut while healing is in progress. Fasting would certainly offer a more convenient way to let the gut rest and heal, but it seems the body requires ongoing energy and nutrients to survive! Soothing nutraceuticals are the mediators between us and our guts. They make the healing process easier by managing any unpleasant symptoms until the gut heals.

- **Slippery elm**: This herb soothes and coats the throat and mouth, but is equally helpful for lining a leaky gut. It creates a slippery blanket that soothes irritation in the gut and offers protection while healing takes place.

  Recommendation: Slippery elm can be taken as a tea, powder, or capsule. There is no standard recommended dosage. Take according to the manufacturer's label.

- **Marshmallow root**: Like slippery elm, marshmallow root dissolves into a slippery substance to create a protective lining inside the gut. It particularly targets the open tight junctions of a leaky gut. This protection allows healing to take place during normal digestion and absorption. It also coats the stomach and is helpful for heartburn and ulcers.

  Recommendation: Marshmallow root can be taken as a tea, liquid, or capsule. There is no standard recommended dosage. Take according to the manufacturer's label.

- **Deglycyrrhizinated licorice (DGL):** DGL is a multifaceted supportive herbal supplement that decreases cortisol levels and rebuilds the mucus lining of the stomach and small intestine to protect from irritating agents. If taken before meals, it prevents abdominal pain, bloating and irritation following a meal.

  Recommendation: 200–300mg taken 30 minutes before each meal. Alternatively, you can sip on licorice tea.

- **Aloe vera:** Like DGL, aloe vera is multifaceted in its healing abilities. It is an anti-inflammatory, has mild antimicrobial properties, and helps clear toxins and irritants from the gut.

  Recommendation: Aloe can be taken as a liquid or capsule. There is no standard recommended dosage. Take according to the manufacturer's label.

- **Quercetin**: Many foods release histamine[h] in the gut, causing an allergic reaction similar to hay fever, and inducing inflammation. Quercetin is a natural antihistamine that stabilizes the cells of the immune system responsible for releasing histamine. Histamine may hinder healing in individuals who respond slowly to other gut-healing nutraceuticals. In these situations, quercetin can help ameliorate these effects and boost the healing process.

Recommendation: 500–1,000mg, taken 2 to 3 times daily.

STEP 3: REPLACE

As we to rebuild the gut and mucosal gut barrier, we must support digestion and absorption. In many cases, an unhealthy gut cannot produce essential digestive enzymes. Hydrochloric acid (HCl) is the primary digestive aid of the stomach. Infections such as *H. pylori*, malnutrition associated with leaky gut, and an overactive immune system reduce the stomach's ability to produce HCl. This acid is critical for protein digestion. In fact, protein will remain in the stomach until HCl adequately digests it. Therefore, insufficient stomach acid results in slow, stagnant protein digestion.

As the protein stays in the stomach, it can putrefy and promote the growth of new infections. If undigested protein leaks from the stomach into the small intestine, it gets absorbed through the loosened junctions of the villi and enters the bloodstream. The body does not recognize undigested protein molecules, so it marks them as foreign objects and the immune system starts an attack. Soon, these foreign proteins become treated as food allergens.

Healthy villi produce specialized digestive enzymes. These enzymes break down the smaller chains of carbohydrates left after the pancreatic enzymes digest the larger carbohydrate chains. The enzymes of the villi act as a fine strainer, catching any carbohydrates that are too big to be deemed safe for the body.

In dysbiosis and leaky gut, many villi are damaged, which hinders their

---

h   Histamine is a substance released by the cells of the immune system in response to allergens and infections. It initiates the inflammatory response and increases blood flow to the area.

ability to produce these specialized enzymes. Larger carbohydrate, fat, and protein pieces slip through the villi, enter the bloodstream, and activate the immune system. Again, the body treats these like food allergens. Are you beginning to understand why an unhealthy gut will cause many false food allergies to appear on an allergy test?

To ensure complete digestion and protect the immune system while healing the gut, you must replace stomach acid (betaine hydrochloric acid or HCl) and digestive enzymes. As healing progresses, the enzyme systems will begin functioning better and digestion will naturally start improving.

Digestive enzymes include:

- **Betaine HCl**: this boosts the production of stomach acid.

  Recommendation: Begin taking 500mg at the beginning of each meal. Monitor bloating and continue to increase dose by 500mg each day until bloating disappears or until you get a warm feeling in your stomach. The average individual may need anywhere from 2,000 to 6,000mg of betaine HCl. High-protein meals will require more betaine HCl than low-protein meals.

- **Broad spectrum digestive enzymes:** these include proteases, lipases, amylase and pepsin.

  Recommendation: Take according to the manufacturer's label (usually 1 or 2 capsules) before each meal.

STEP 4: REINOCULATE

The final step of the "4R" plan focuses on rebuilding the protective mucosal gut barrier by reinoculating it with beneficial bacteria. These bacteria create the thick, protective mucus layer that acts as the first line of defense in the gut.

Dysbiosis and SIBO often precede leaky gut, so beneficial bacteria must take back their home to correct these conditions. As we apply the first step of the "4R" plan (Remove) and kill the yeast and dangerous bacteria, we are evicting the unwanted guests from our gut. But unless we reinoculate with beneficial bacteria, the bad guys will eventually take over again.

The beneficial bacteria are probiotics ("pro-" means good, and "-biota" means bacteria). Probiotics include various strains of bacteria that work together to rebuild the mucosal gut barrier and carry out their defense roles.

Probiotics take time to colonize in the gut and often need a significant amount of nurturing. Therefore, we use various methods of supplying these vital bacteria and encouraging their growth.

- **High-quality probiotics:** It is important to choose a supplement that includes multiple strains of bacteria such as lactobacilli, bifidobacteria, and acidophilus. Probiotics are live bacteria and should be stored in the refrigerator for optimal survival. Some brands claim to be shelf stable, but it is still a good idea to store them in a cold environment. It is also important to make sure the capsules are acid-resistant so the bacteria will survive the hydrochloric acid of the stomach. Remember, most commercial probiotics don't contain enough cultures to reinoculate the gut successfully.

  Recommendation: 25–75 billion CFU each night before bed.

- **Fermented Foods:** Fermented foods such as sauerkraut, kimchi, kombucha, water kefir, kvass, and fermented vegetables are excellent ways of gaining small amounts of probiotics with each meal. Fermented foods are economical, easy to make, tasty, and support the supplemental probiotics. You can find instructions and resources for making fermented foods in the Resource section of this book.

  Recommendation: At least ¼ cup of fermented veggies each day.

- **Prebiotics:** Prebiotics are fibrous foods that feed probiotics and help them grow in the gut. Prebiotics are soluble fibers including arabinogalactan, oligosaccharides, inulin, and fructooligosaccharides (FOS). They are components of apples, onions, garlic, asparagus, Jerusalem artichokes, and leeks. Some probiotic supplements include prebiotic fibers.

Recommendation: There is no specific recommendation, but include prebiotic foods in your meal every day.

Caution: Some individuals with advanced cases of SIBO and IBS may not be able to consume supplemental prebiotics or prebiotic foods without experiencing significant abdominal bloating and pain. In these cases, I suggest taking herbal antimicrobials for several months to reduce the microbial load before introducing prebiotics.

DEALING WITH THE DIE-OFF REACTION

When beginning any detox or healing program that involves killing microorganisms, you must be prepared to feel worse before you feel better. Symptoms will intensify as the dying organisms release their toxins. This reaction is called the "die-off" reaction, or more technically, the Herxheimer ("herx") reaction. View this as a positive sign of progress and use it as a motivation to keep moving forward. Instead of indicating that the plan is not working, the herx reaction is actually proof the plan is working correctly.

The herx reaction feels like the flu. Fever, chills, achiness, fatigue, brain fog, and gastrointestinal symptoms are common signs of die-off issues. Sometimes, skin rashes, nasal congestion, or allergies can get worse as well.

Die-off symptoms occur when the toxins released from dying microorganisms accumulate faster than the body's detoxification organs (liver, kidney, bowels) can eliminate them. As they increase in the blood, various organ systems get flooded with toxins. Individuals with larger quantities of microorganisms, or higher toxin loads in their body, will experience more severe herx reactions. Therefore, herx reactions can be a good indicator of the body's detoxification ability and its current toxin load.

Most herx reactions pass within a few days; however, if you have a severe case of dysbiosis, you may have to decrease the antimicrobial agents and allow your normal detoxification processes to "catch up." It isn't healthy to expose your body to a flood of toxins and expect it to heal. Therefore, if the die-off reactions do not pass within a few days or are severe, you will need to take the journey more slowly.

Here are some helpful tips for dealing with herx reactions, making the journey a bit more tolerable:

- **Drink a lot of liquid!** Adequate hydration is essential for diluting toxins and speeding their elimination through the kidneys and colon. Lemon water is an excellent option because it hydrates, alkalinizes, and provides extra vitamin C.

- **Take buffered vitamin C.** Vitamin C is a potent antioxidant. Antioxidants help neutralize the harmful free radicals generated by toxins that can damage surrounding cells. Large doses of buffered ascorbic acid (vitamin C) help protect healthy cells from damaging toxins. Many people can only tolerate larger doses of vitamin C if it is buffered with potassium and magnesium. Take 2 to 4 grams of buffered vitamin C in divided doses throughout the day.

- **Get quality sleep.** Rest is essential when the body is burdened with toxins. Adults must aim for 7 to 9 hours of sleep each night to restore all the vital body systems and aid in healing. Ideally, you should sleep from 10 p.m. to 6 a.m. for optimal adrenal restoration.

- **Improve the lymphatic system with rebounding and dry skin brushing**. Most toxins get filtered out of the blood through the lymphatic system. If the lymph is stagnant, toxins accumulate, leading to a herx reaction. Rebounding on a mini trampoline for five minutes each day is an easy way to encourage lymphatic drainage, while dry body brushing will stimulate better lymphatic flow. To dry brush, purchase a stiff-bristled body brush. Starting with your extremities, brush your skin in long strokes toward your groin and armpits, where your lymph nodes are concentrated. Dry brushing is best performed before a shower.

- **Address constipation**. The liver delivers large loads of toxins to the gut, expecting it to quickly eliminate them through the colon. It is imperative to maintain regular bowel movements each day for detoxification. If toxins remain in the colon, they get reabsorbed into the bloodstream and increase the body's toxin load. Magnesium encourages regular bowel movements. Taking 500 to 1,000mg every night will not only stimulate a morning bowel movement but will also relax your muscles so you can sleep better.

- **Take Epsom salt bath**s. Epsom salts supply magnesium sulfate in the way our body can most readily absorb it: through the skin. Magnesium is helpful for elimination and sleep, alkalinizing the body and neutralizing toxins by enhancing detoxification. Use 2 cups of Epsom salts in a full tub of bathwater, two to three times each week.

- **Reduce antimicrobials**. In some cases, if the above support measures aren't effective, it is necessary to lower the dose of antimicrobials you are taking to remove harmful organisms and proceed at a slower pace. A toxic body is not a healing body.

In the remaining chapters of Part 2, we will explore the nutritional plan for healing the gut. We will review each food group and discover which foods heal and which ones impede the process. These chapters are an extension of the "Remove" part of the "4R" plan, which involves removing food allergens, inflammatory foods, and foods that feed gut infections.

Chapter Summary: Healing the gut is essential for reversing disease and chronic illness. The "4R" plan focuses on removing triggers, repairing the gut, replacing digestive support, and reinoculating the gut with good bacteria. Over time, the tight junctions will close, the villi get rebuilt, and the protective mucosal gut barrier is restored. As we balance the microbial environment of the gut, the body is better protected, the immune system calms, and we reduce systemic inflammation. Collectively, these actions reverse disease processes and reduce your risks for developing chronic illness.

CHAPTER 12:

SUGARS & SWEETENERS

WE BEGIN OUR INVESTIGATION INTO a healing diet with the food group that is the most destructive to our gut, and which spearheads dysbiosis, SIBO, and leaky gut. Many may wish we could skip this chapter altogether. Just remember that although sometimes ignorance is bliss, disease is not arrested by its presence. Therefore, I want to explore the raw facts about sugar and sweeteners, because these are among the worst culprits in promoting disease and chronic illness.

SUGAR IS ADDICTIVE

You don't simply have a "sweet tooth." It's not just a monthly chocolate buzz for women. We all love sugar. I love sugar, too.

Over the past several decades, however, our sugar consumption has grown exponentially and today, sugar is a societal addiction. Perhaps, it is one of the most prevalent and dangerous because it isn't selective in choosing its victims. It imprisons children, adults, the elite, and the impoverished alike. Everyone.

Very few people willingly acknowledge the addictive nature of sugar. Policy makers turn their heads in fear that such a revelation might lead to a public outcry or demand for food manufacturers to reformulate their recipes. However unpleasant and inconvenient, the facts remain. Sugar can be as addictive as cocaine and opioids. An article published in July 2013 in *Current Opinion in Clinical Nutrition and Metabolic Care* states the following:

Available evidence in humans shows that sugar and sweetness can induce reward and craving that are comparable in magnitude to those induced by addictive drugs. Although this evidence is limited by the inherent difficulty of comparing different types of rewards and psychological experiences in humans, it is nevertheless supported by recent experimental research on sugar and sweet reward in laboratory rats. Overall, this research has revealed that sugar and sweet reward can not only substitute addictive drugs, like cocaine, but can even be more rewarding and attractive. At the neurobiological level, the neural substrates of sugar and sweet reward appear to be more robust than those of cocaine.[66]

Also, consider the following from a review published in a 2008 edition of *Neuroscience & Biobehavioral Reviews*:

The experimental question is whether or not sugar can be a substance of abuse and lead to a natural form of addiction... Sugar is noteworthy as a substance that releases opioids and dopamine and thus might be expected to have addictive potential. This review summarizes evidence of sugar dependence in an animal model. Four components of addiction are analyzed. "Bingeing," "withdrawal," "craving," and cross-sensitization are each given operational definitions and demonstrated behaviorally with sugar bingeing as the reinforcer. These behaviors are then related to neurochemical changes in the brain that also occur with addictive drugs... The evidence supports the hypothesis that under certain circumstances rats can become sugar dependent. This may translate to some human conditions as suggested by the literature on eating disorders and obesity.[67]

Most disturbing is the reality that this addiction may begin the moment we start to eat food. Sweetened foods such as jarred baby food, teething wafers, Cheerios, Happy Meals, and Lunchables tantalize our children's taste buds. These early habits strongly influence the future health of our children, including their risk for obesity.

SUGAR'S HEALTH CONSEQUENCES

The food industry and government agencies try to deny it, but research suggests our beloved sugar is a contributing agent in the following conditions:[68]

- Obesity

- Diabetes

- Cardiovascular disease

- High cholesterol

- Cancer

- Autoimmunity issues

- Alzheimer's disease (now considered type 3 diabetes[69])

- Behavioral conditions

- Mood conditions

- Cognitive decline

- Non-alcoholic fatty liver disease

- Inflammatory conditions

The association between sugar and our health is rooted in two mechanisms. First, sugar is highly inflammatory. It initiates inflammation in the gut and, consequently, throughout the entire body. Sugar is strongly correlated to the obesity epidemic. As fat cells begin growing and accumulating in the body, they release copious amounts of inflammatory factors. These intensify systemic inflammation and give rise to various chronic health conditions, including diabetes and cardiovascular disease. If we reduced or eliminated sugar in our diets, we would see a corresponding decrease in obesity and experience fewer chronic inflammatory conditions.

Secondly, sugar feeds yeast and harmful bacteria in the gut, inducing dysbiosis, SIBO, leaky gut, and systemic inflammation. As we learned earlier, systemic inflammation begins in the gut and becomes the foundation of many chronic health conditions. If sugar sets this train in motion, then eliminating sugar is a big step in bringing it to a stop.

SUGAR CONSUMPTION

Despite the evidence against sugar, our consumption continues to escalate wildly with no signs of stopping. Part of the problem is that we can't recognize the forms and chemical ingredients in which sugar is being disguised. Processed foods are the chief sources of excess sugars, with breakfast cereals and sweetened beverages being the worst culprits.[70] In the 2009–2010 National Health and Nutrition Examination Survey (NHANES), 89.7 percent of the energy (calories) in processed foods came from added sugars, and 82.1 percent of Americans exceeded the recommended limits for added sugar consumption.[71] Finally, the September 2013 report from Credit Suisse's Research Institute gave an alarming report that "30–40% of health care expenditures in the USA go to help address issues that are closely tied to the excess consumption of sugar." They estimated that our sugar addiction costs approximately $1 trillion in health care costs each year.[72]

THE BOTTOM LINE FOR GUT HEALING

The first "R" (Remove) in the "4R" plan indicates we must eliminate inflammatory foods, as well as foods that feed yeast and bacteria. Sugar sits at the top of the list.

To fully eliminate sugar, we must learn how to recognize it and replace it with better options. Let's look at three considerations that can help us determine which sweeteners are safe and which are dangerous.

1. How quickly does the sweetener break down into glucose or fructose, or is it already in these forms? The faster a sugar turns into glucose or fructose, the more efficiently it feeds sizable amounts of yeast and bacteria. And the quicker sugar becomes glucose, the faster it enters the bloodstream and induces inflammation. Glucose is easy to spot on a food label, and all types of "sugar" (white sugar, brown sugar, cane sugar, etc.) contain at least 50 percent glucose and 50 percent fructose. Fructose doesn't absorb into the bloodstream quickly because the gut lacks sufficient receptors for it. Therefore, it remains in the gut, feeding yeast and bacteria. Sources of pure glucose and fructose, or sugars that turn into glucose quickly, must be *completely* eliminated.

2. Is the sweetener bound to fiber? Building upon the previous consideration, sugars linked to fiber do not turn into glucose quickly because digestive enzymes must work to unbind them. These sugar sources are less likely to provide a feast for yeast and bacteria and will not flood the bloodstream with glucose, causing an inflammatory eruption. Most natural sources of sugar such as fruit contain this sugar/fiber duo. However, they still supply glucose and therefore, must be used *sparingly*.

3. Does the sweetener have any caloric value? Calories are measurements of energy from molecules such as glucose and fructose. Some sweeteners may taste sweet, but do not have any glucose or fructose molecules, so they can't feed yeast or bacteria and certainly won't raise your blood sugar. These are safe sweeteners if they come from natural plant sources. Chemically produced noncaloric sweeteners are health catastrophes. As part of a gut-healing diet, plant-based, noncaloric sweeteners are the *only* safe sweeteners.

ELIMINATE COMPLETELY

- Any ingredient that ends in "–ose"
- Any ingredient that states it is a "sugar"
- Any ingredient that states it is a "syrup"
- Any ingredient that states it is a "juice"
- Sucanat, honey, agave, malt, molasses, and maltodextrin

USE SPARINGLY

- Coconut palm sugar
- Coconut syrup
- Palm sugar
- Fresh fruits
- Yacon

NOTE: Some individuals with advanced cases of *Candida* infections, dysbiosis, SIBO, or leaky gut should eliminate this category for at least six months. Those with less severe gut challenges may tolerate very small amounts, but no more than once each week.

SAFE SWEETENERS

- Stevia

- Monkfruit

- Erythritol

- Xylitol

Sweeteners with the "-ol" suffix are sugar alcohols. They don't contain glucose, but they can cause bloating and abdominal pain in some individuals, and especially those with SIBO or IBS. It is important to monitor symptoms while using these and to only use them sparingly.

If you aren't sensitive to sugar alcohols, xylitol (birch sugar) may impart some health benefits. Many individuals are aware of xylitol's positive effects on oral health, but it can also offset one of the carcinogenic[i] byproducts of yeast fermentation, released into the gut when yeast feeds off sugars.[73]

COMMERCIAL NONCALORIC SUGAR SUBSTITUTES

Commercial noncaloric sugar substitutes are even more dangerous than white sugar. Chemists discovered most of these chemical sweeteners by accident. The FDA approved them through illegitimate practices including bribery, "behind the door" exchanges, and conflicts of interest. The so-called studies the FDA uses to verify their safety are deceptive, if not outright false, and performed by the very companies that manufacture these sweeteners. Independent studies tell a very different story about their safety—or lack thereof.

The noncaloric sweeteners I am referring to include:

- Aspartame (NutraSweet, Equal)

- Sucralose (Splenda)

- Saccharin (Sweet'N Low)

---

i   Cancer-causing

- Acesulfame-K (often found in diet sodas)

Aspartame is the most common sugar substitute, so we will focus on this ingredient as a prototype for other noncaloric sugar substitutes.

When the body metabolizes aspartame, it produces the following three molecules:

1. **Phenylalanine**: An amino acid that stimulates excitatory neurotransmitters in the brain at doses supplied by aspartame. This stimulatory action makes aspartame addictive because it gives a "high" similar to street drugs.

2. **Aspartic acid**: An amino acid that lowers serotonin (our "good mood" hormone) and contributes to depression at the high doses supplied by aspartame.

3. **Methanol**: An alcohol that converts to formaldehyde in the liver—yes, the same product used to preserve the dead. Delicious, huh? Formaldehyde is the most dangerous component of aspartame because the body can't excrete it. Instead, it stores it in your fat cells. Levels accumulate and increase the body's toxin load.

To our horror, the FDA thinks small amounts of aspartame have negligible health implications. But considering all the food products that contain aspartame (sugar-free gum, vitamins, diet drinks, sugar-free foods, etc.), we could be getting a hefty cumulative dose without realizing it. The FDA fails to tell us how much aspartame we can consume before it becomes dangerous to our health. Of course, a toxin is toxic in any amount.

Documented adverse side effects from aspartame surpass those of any other food additive. The most commonly reported side effect is headaches, but you can find a laundry list of adverse effects in the government's database of reported adverse effects of food additives. Many of these include neurological side effects that affect cognition and mood.[74] Perhaps the most dangerous outcome of regular aspartame consumption is increased risk for cancer.[75]

Those wishing to lose weight are the most frequent consumers of aspartame-laden food products. It's an ironic situation, because aspartame accomplishes the opposite. Aspartame fools the brain into believing you consumed sugar when you didn't. The brain responds by telling the pancreas to produce and secrete insulin to lower the "sugar" in the blood. Insulin unlocks your cells' ability to absorb glucose from the bloodstream, but the expected glucose isn't there. Instead, the cells absorb the small amounts of free-floating glucose that are continually present to provide energy to the brain. As your normal blood sugar drops, the body faces a state of crisis. It responds by giving signals to eat, and so you eat. A low blood sugar level often triggers you to eat high-glucose foods that quickly raise the blood sugar. Ultimately, you will consume more calories because the "diet trick" didn't work.

In summary, chemical noncaloric sugar substitutes should never be a part of a healthy diet, regardless of your gut's health.

SUGAR CRAVINGS

I feel it is important to warn anyone embarking on the journey of gut healing to prepare for some intense sugar cravings in the initial stages of the "4R" plan. The abundance of yeast and bacteria in the gut will send strong signals to the brain seeking sugar. Sugar is their primary food source, and as the brain interprets these messages, you will experience intense sugar cravings. Stand firm, knowing the cravings will pass; as you restore the health of your gut, you will establish a desire for healthy foods. As the antimicrobial herbals decrease the populations of yeast and bacteria, the cravings will subside. Much to your surprise, broccoli will sound better than a refined white bagel or candy bar because it will satiate without taking you for a ride on the blood sugar roller coaster.

I understand that some of you may feel as though I am suggesting the permanent elimination of all pleasurable foods. Rest assured, this is not the case! Sugar won't always be a problem. As you heal your gut, your relationship with sugar will become healthier and an occasional indulgence won't send your health on a downward spiral. Each year, I enjoy a sugar-laden piece of chocolate cheesecake on my birthday without guilt. Similarly, when I visit friends or family, I don't turn up my nose at their offer of dessert. I enjoy these occasional treats knowing that my routine food choices nourish my gut and my body.

Remember, the "4R" plan is a journey to heal your gut, but at the end of the journey, you will discover that you have developed healthier habits to maintain your state of health. It is at this finish line that you can enjoy a balanced diet that includes occasional treats.

Chapter Summary: Sugar and sweeteners feed yeast and unhealthy bacteria and trigger inflammation. Therefore, we must remove most sugars and sweeteners from a gut-healing plan. Stevia is the best option as a sweetener.

CHAPTER 13:

GRAINS & GLUTEN

G RAINS ARE THE NEXT MOST influential food group to impact gut health. The reason is simple: grain becomes glucose when digested, so the result of consuming grains is similar to that of sugar. Some of the redeeming qualities associated with grains are the presence of fiber, vitamins, protein, and some fats.

REFINED VS. WHOLE GRAINS

Grain has become a significant part of our diet since agribusiness, and the growing subsidy programs supporting it, convinced the USDA to place grain at the base of the American food pyramid, declaring it to be the foundation of our diet. Politicians hid their agendas (the promotion of grains) behind the auspices of new national food guidelines.

As years passed and government subsidy programs continued to grow, it became imperative to devise ways of decreasing the cost of food. Industrialization introduced a plethora of food additives and processed "food" products constructed from a few mass-produced grains: corn, soy, and wheat. As the demand for these crops grew, scientists discovered how to refine and genetically modify them. The purpose of this new technology was to produce greater yields, extend the shelf life and uses of grains, and expand our pocketbooks.

Sadly, most consumers don't realize the grain consumed today is radically different from its original state. Eighty percent of our processed foods are made from refined, genetically modified grain. It is this "new" style of grain that is largely responsible for our damaged guts and deteriorating health.

To understand the difference between refined and unrefined grain, let's look at the anatomy of grain.

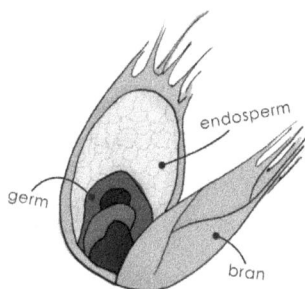

Kernel of Grain

The process of refining removes the following components from grain:

- Bran: contains fiber, B vitamins, and minerals
- Germ: contains B vitamins, vitamin E, minerals, and phytonutrients

The starchy endosperm remains and is the foundation for making white flour, white rice, quick oats, and all processed grain products like pasta, cereal, crackers, and more. Refined grain is convenient for the food industry because it increases the food product's shelf life. The oils and fat-soluble vitamins (vitamin E) can oxidize and become rancid with time when exposed to air and light. Removing these nutrients increases shelf life, but it also decreases the nutritional value of the grain.

After the surge of refined grain swept through America, we began witnessing malnutrition in many of our children. Research pointed the finger at our heavy intake of nutrient-deficient, refined grain. Hence, the process of enriching grain with lost vitamins was born. However, one problem remains. Enriched grains only contain a fraction of the vitamins they possessed in their original, whole-grain state.

Another problem with refined grain is that it lacks prebiotic fiber, necessary to feed healthy bacteria in the gut. Instead, the starch-filled endosperm becomes pure glucose, which not only feeds yeast and harmful bacteria but also raises our blood sugar quickly. Together, this promotes dysbiosis, SIBO, leaky gut, and systemic inflammation. It begs the question of which came first: our discovery of health conditions linked to systemic inflammation, or the explosion of refined grain? Once the food market was saturated with inexpensive, refined grain products, we no longer desired the vegetables, fruits, nuts, seeds, beans, and legumes that once created the foundation of our diet.

It is also interesting to note that as of the mid-1990s, most refined grain is genetically modified to tolerate greater amounts of herbicides and insecticides. So not only are refined grains stripped of nutrition, feeding dysbiosis and inflammation, but they also impart traces of toxic chemicals and genetically modified organisms.

Because refined grain plays a significant role in establishing dysbiosis, its elimination from our diet is vital for healing the gut. Whole grains are also questionable, but we will cover this issue later. Before we do, let's consider another highly controversial, hot-button topic that impacts gut health: gluten.

GLUTEN

Gluten is often a health problem. Unfortunately, being "gluten-free" has become trendy among uninformed consumers and is increasingly exploited by food manufacturers, complicating and discrediting the seriousness of this issue.

Gluten is the protein found in wheat, rye, and barley. Oats, although they don't naturally contain gluten, can carry gluten contaminants from being processed on the same equipment used to process glutenous grains.

Celiac Disease

The medical community first recognized gluten as a potential health issue after discovering the dangerous autoimmune condition known as celiac disease, or celiac sprue. If someone with this condition consumes even a trace of gluten, their immune system immediately attacks and destroys the villi. The intestinal wall becomes almost entirely void of villi, which leads to an extremely leaky and inflamed gut. A dangerous state of malnutrition soon develops. Celiac disease is considered a genetic autoimmune condition affecting approximately 1 percent of the world.[76] But wait! If celiac disease only affects 1 percent of the world, why does nearly 30 percent of the public claim to have improved health with a gluten-free diet?[77]

Non-Celiac Gluten Sensitivity

As more people report significant health improvements after eliminating gluten, despite the absence of true celiac disease, researchers are scrambling to find answers. Another persistent condition known as non-celiac gluten sensitivity is quickly emerging.[78] The prevalence of this condition is exponentially greater than that of celiac disease and may explain why so many individuals find relief from eliminating gluten. Symptoms of non-celiac gluten sensitivity are similar to those of celiac disease, but a definitive autoimmune reaction is missing, as well as the severity of symptoms that characterize celiac disease. In both cases, dysbiosis and leaky gut are present, but celiac disease can quickly become life-threatening, whereas non-celiac gluten sensitivity has a slower and less noticeable impact on health.

Zonulin and Wheat Lectins

Even if we don't notice negative symptoms associated with consuming gluten, zonulin should give us reason to reconsider our attitude toward gluten.

Nearly a decade ago, researchers sought to understand how gluten affects gut permeability. They recognized its role in destroying villi and tight junctions in celiac disease. But what about the rest of the population that didn't carry the genetic susceptibility to celiac disease, yet seemed to experience resolution of common gut conditions after eliminating gluten? Slowly, research began to put the pieces together.[79, 80]

When gluten enters the intestine, special receptors on the surface of the villi recognize a component of gluten known as gliadin. Gliadin is an antagonistic instigator. It "tickles" these particular receptors on the villi, causing them to release a molecule called zonulin. Zonulin opens the tight junctions of the small intestine and causes the gut lining to become permeable, or leaky. This response isn't limited to a select group of people—everyone who was tested showed this response to gliadin. You may be wondering why so many people eat gluten and don't complain of symptoms associated with leaky gut. Here's the caveat: our personal genetics determine how much zonulin our villi release in response to gliadin. Those with the genetic susceptibility to celiac will produce a lot of zonulin, creating a very leaky gut. Everyone secretes varying amounts of zonulin in response to gliadin, and therefore, we don't all experiences the same degree of "leakiness" from consuming gluten.

Not only is gliadin responsible for causing a leaky gut, but it can change the actions of our immune system. Gliadin can activate T cells and prompt the innate immune system to launch an inflammatory response. These activities aren't limited to those with celiac disease, but are shared by everyone who consumes gluten.[81]

Gluten also carries a group of components known as lectins. These serve to protect the grain from insects and fungi while it is growing. Lectins are like a built-in pesticide. They may be advantageous for the plant, but they aren't helpful to the digestive and immune systems. Lectins resist digestive enzymes and heat. They also like to attach to the cells of the intestine, where they are recognized as foreign invaders and attacked by the immune system. All plant foods have lectins, including beans, legumes, nuts, and seeds, but the lectins associated with gluten are zealous and can also bind to other organ tissues, inducing inflammation around those organs.[82] Gluten lectins provide one explanation for gluten's association with pancreas destruction and thyroid problems.

Wheat lectin also acts like zonulin and can increase intestinal permeability while it is attached to the intestinal cells. It fosters the development of leaky gut. Soaking grain removes some lectin, which is why this practice has become popular among health advocates, but for those with poor gut health, complete avoidance is the best solution for healing.

Unfortunately, no one is exempt from gluten's power to release zonulin, open the tight junctions of the intestine, activate the immune system, and induce systemic inflammation. In some particularly susceptible individuals, it may even harm other organs.

If you are experiencing dysbiosis, SIBO, inflammation, and a weakened immune system, you should not discount the effects of gluten. Nutrient availability and immune activation can control our genetic expression by turning genes on and off. Therefore, a poor diet coupled with an active immune system can make you more sensitive to the effects of gluten. Gluten is considered a potential trigger for autoimmune conditions because of its ability to control our genetic expression. For example, if you have a genetic predisposition for rheumatoid arthritis, gluten can work with the immune system to "turn on" the expression of this gene, giving you an active case of this autoimmune condition.[83] Gluten can become a trigger for anyone with compromised health, and we must remove all dietary triggers if we want to heal our gut.

Some people ask if organic and sprouted wheat are superior, or nonproblematic, sources of gluten, suggesting that these do not elicit the adverse health effects associated with our more modern wheat. It is true that recent agricultural changes have delivered a wheat kernel vastly different from its ancient ancestor. Gliadin has undergone several genetic transformations since the mid-1900s as farmers have selectively bred to increase yields. Selective breeding is not the same as the genetic engineering that produces GMOs, although there are some similarities. Selective breeding uses genes from different specimens of the same species to enhance that species' characteristics, while GMOs are a combination of genetic material from different species that wouldn't breed in nature. By the late 1990s, nearly all wheat had been genetically transformed into a new variety. Modern wheat contains double the amount of chromosomes compared to ancient wheat, which also increases the gliadin content. Greater concentrations of gliadin can explain the recent explosion of gut problems associated with gluten.

Modern wheat production introduced another issue for our gut as well. Natural wheat matures at different times, but in the agricultural industry, this is not convenient. Farmers discovered that by applying glyphosate (Roundup) near the end of the crop season, maturation would speed up to provide a greater yield of wheat at harvest. Unfortunately, this practice leaves residues of glyphosate on the harvested wheat. This toxic herbicide has been implicated in numerous health conditions, including our declining tolerance to gluten. Interestingly, this practice was established in the late 1990s, right when we began noting an increase in gut issues.

Organic wheat may keep you safe from glyphosate, but organic, sprouted, cracked, crushed, soaked wheat has still been selectively bred to contain increased levels of gliadin, and this component still increases zonulin and promotes a leaky gut.

GLUTEN-FREE GRAINS

So far, we have established that whole grain is better than refined grain, and gluten-free grain is better than glutenous grain. Now let's talk about the issue of consuming grains in any form, at any time.

There are many fine gluten-free whole grains on the market, which we will look at shortly, but before we do, I want you to consider whether grain in any form supports or hinders healing.

Whole grain can supply fiber, minerals, and vitamins, but its starch content is high. We are still providing a glucose source for yeast and unhealthy bacteria to grow in our gut. In fact, one reason we love bread is that it temporarily makes the yeast and bacteria happy. They send "happy" signals to our brain, which associates glucose with feelings of satisfaction.

All grains contain the built-in pesticide lectin. Different types of grains contain distinct forms of lectins, but each can irritate the immune system and instigate an inflammatory reaction. Some grains contain additional nutrients that fight inflammation and neutralize the negative reaction. However, the immune system is almost always active in an unhealthy gut, and small triggers can aggravate the situation.

Due to its starchy interior, grain forces the pancreas to release insulin in response to the glucose. Insulin is an inflammatory hormone, and controlling it is paramount for optimal health. Alternative starch sources such as vegetables and beans contain more fiber and antioxidants to counteract the effects of insulin. Grain doesn't provide the quantity of fiber and antioxidants that other food groups supply to mitigate the effects of insulin.

To better understand how grain consumption affects insulin, let's consider a recent study. This study sought to determine the consequences of a paleo (grain-free) diet or a Mediterranean diet (which includes a moderate amount of whole grains) on insulin levels and risk factors for diabetes.[84, 85] After 10 days, the test group consuming the grain-free paleo diet experienced a reduction in blood pressure, insulin levels, cholesterol, and triglycerides, and their cells responded to insulin more efficiently. After 15 months, the inflammatory factors of the test group were reduced by 82 percent after consuming a grain-free paleo diet, compared to the group that consumed the whole grain-based Mediterranean diet and still showed immune activity.

If our goal is to reduce inflammation and calm the immune system, any form of grain may not be advantageous for healing. Individuals with less severe cases of dysbiosis, SIBO, or leaky gut may tolerate small portions of grains while continuing to see progress in their healing journey. If you are one of these individuals, only consume gluten-free whole grains. Ideally, these should be soaked to reduce the lectin content.

PSEUDO-GRAINS OR NON-GRAINS

A unique group of pseudo-grains exists and has contributed to the controversy over grains. These plants aren't technically grains because they don't belong to the grass family. Rather, they are seeds with grain-like characteristics. Here are a few examples of pseudo-grains:

- Amaranth
- Buckwheat
- Quinoa
- Millet
- Teff
- Wild rice

Pseudo-grains contain smaller quantities of lectins, but they also possess anti-nutrients, which are compounds found in beans, legumes, nuts and seeds. They interfere with the absorption of vitamins and minerals. Unlike authentic grains, pseudo-grains have higher levels of protein, antioxidants, vitamins, and minerals, which may nullify their lectins and anti-nutrients, making them an acceptable choice for gut healing. Like gluten-free grains, your individual reactions and circumstances must control the decision of whether to eat them. Pseudo-grains are certainly the best option to include in a gut-healing diet if you choose to consume grains at all.

THE BOTTOM LINE FOR GUT HEALING

Unfortunately, there isn't a one-size-fits-all answer to this complicated food group, but there are some general guidelines everyone should follow to heal the gut. Any gray areas (noted below) will require a proper evaluation of your current condition with a knowledgeable practitioner, or individual trial and error.

Everyone should eliminate all grains and pseudo-grains for at least 30 days when beginning the "4R" plan. The purpose is to remove all potential triggers to the immune system, allowing it to rest. Once healing begins, some individuals can tolerate small quantities of pseudo-grains, but should have no more than one to two small servings each day. As healing progresses (usually after six months), occasional servings of gluten-free whole grains and flours are acceptable for most people.

ELIMINATE COMPLETELY

- All gluten: wheat (spelt, bulgur, couscous, farro, durum, kamut, semolina, graham), barley, rye, non-gluten-free-certified oats, and triticale
- All refined, processed (i.e., white) grains: white rice, white flours, etc.

USE SPARINGLY

- Gluten-free whole grains: brown rice, corn, certified GF oats, sorghum
- Grain flours: millet flour, teff flour, corn flour, rice flour, oat flour, sorghum flour

What's the big deal with flours? Although they contain the whole grain, processing separates the starch from the bran, making it easily digestible. Glucose quickly accumulates as enzymes digest the starch, increasing your blood sugar and forcing the pancreas to release more insulin. Therefore, flours are more inflammatory than the whole grain.

SAFE PSEUDO-GRAINS

- Amaranth

- Buckwheat

- Quinoa

- Millet

- Teff

- Wild rice

Chapter Summary: Gluten and refined grains feed yeast and bacteria, contributing to the development of dysbiosis, SIBO, and, eventually, a leaky gut. Gluten also triggers leaky gut by provoking the secretion of zonulin, a compound that "opens up" tight junctions. All grains contain lectins that activate the immune system, promote inflammation, and cause gut distress. Therefore, many choose to eliminate grains altogether when repairing the gut. Pseudo-grains are grain-like seeds that may provide a safer option for some people.

CHAPTER 14:

DAIRY

Dairy products are not helpful for healing the gut, based on several compounding issues that we will briefly consider.

ANTIBIOTICS, HORMONES, INFLAMMATORY FATS, AND PROTEINS

The quality of our modern dairy products is significantly inferior to that of previous generations. In the 1950s, high-volume commercial animal farms, known as Concentrated Animal Feeding Operations (CAFOs), began displacing small family farms. The face of both the meat and dairy industry changed. Today, scores of cows live their lives in crowded stalls, fed unnatural diets of genetically modified grains littered with plastics and animal byproducts. They are routinely impregnated to maintain a high milk output, and the stress they experience limits their lifespan to less than four years. Various diseases and mastitis are inevitable. A steady diet of growth hormones increases milk production by nearly six times and antibiotics are given to keep disease at bay.

As with humans, drugs and toxins given to cows are stored in fat and transferred to the milk of lactating animals. We feel compelled to place warning labels on prescription drugs to deter lactating mothers from potentially harming their infants. And yet it's acceptable to give dairy cows massive amounts of hormones and antibiotics and sell the milk to the entire human population. Laboratory analyses confirms the presence of hormones and drugs in our milk supply, which contributes to our increasing health problems such as antibiotic resistance, gut conditions, and hormone imbalances.[86]

Commercial milk lacks the healthy nutrients that once distinguished it as a nutritious beverage in the past. When cows graze on green pasture, the milk they produce contains anti-inflammatory omega-3 fats; conjugated linoleic acid (CLA); and vitamins D, E, and A. Conversely, milk produced by commercial, grain-fed cows lacks these nutrients and has higher levels of inflammatory saturated and trans fats.

Grass-fed cows have stronger immune systems that impart immune-boosting immunoglobulins (antibodies) in their milk. Commercial grain-fed cows lack these compounds in their milk and burden our immune system with inflammatory fats, drug residues, and damaged proteins.

Homogenization and pasteurization deplete milk of many heat-sensitive nutrients such as antioxidants and vitamins D, A, and E. During pasteurization, the heat applied to kill bacteria also disturbs delicate protein chains, leaving them damaged and potentially dangerous. Many researchers have raised the possibility that homogenization (the process of blending the cream into the milk) creates incredibly small fat molecules that may trigger various health conditions such as cardiovascular disease.

Obtaining raw milk and dairy products from exclusively pastured (grass-fed) cows can eliminate the issues of drug residues, inflammatory fats, nutrient depletion, and dangerous proteins. But as concerning as these issues are, they are not the sole reason dairy is a poor choice for gut healing.

CASEIN

Dairy is unquestionably one of the most common food allergies. This fact may come as a surprise, considering the prevalence of dairy in our food. The problem is that dairy is often a latent allergen, delaying its symptoms. Therefore, it is often an unrecognized allergy. Colic, sinusitis, ear infections, eczema, congestion, asthma, GERD (gastroesophageal reflux disease), and ADHD are often expressions of a latent dairy allergy. Casein is the offending component. It comprises 80 percent of the protein in dairy; whey supplies the other 20 percent.

An allergic reaction to casein is most prominent in infants and children because their digestive systems are immature. The casein protein of cow's milk is much larger than the protein of human milk. It is, after all, designed to nourish large calves rather than small human babies.

Compounding this issue are various intolerances to a specific component of milk, such as casein, whey, or lactose. An intolerance causes symptoms that are milder than those of an allergy. Allergies involve a direct attack on the offender by the immune system, causing more severe symptoms. An intolerance may not require direct immune activity, or its involvement is minimal, explaining the mild symptoms.

With the rise of dairy allergies and intolerances, researchers are identifying many associations between dairy components and gastrointestinal health. For example, the A1 variant of the casein protein found in common cattle breeds increases gut motility, activates pain receptors in the gut, and increases inflammatory factors.[87] Gut symptoms remain the most notorious expression of a dairy intolerance. Casein's ability to trigger a low-grade inflammatory response on the gut's surface is at the core of this situation.[88]

As a final note for those who advocate raw milk as a better option: it *is* a better option for healthy individuals who tolerate dairy because it contains live enzymes that aid in its digestibility. But it remains a poor choice for healing the gut. Casein, the inflammatory component of milk, is the same protein regardless of whether it originates from raw or commercial milk. Fermenting the milk does not eliminate it, either. Casein is a component of all dairy, and most often, it is the offender in cases of allergy or intolerance.

GOAT AND SHEEP MILK

Some people who are allergic or intolerant to cow milk can tolerate goat and sheep milk. Casein is present in all milk and can still present a problem to sensitive individuals, but the type of casein in sheep and goat milk is less inflammatory. Beta-casein is the dominant protein in sheep and goat milk. Cow milk contains more alpha-casein, which is far more inflammatory compared to beta-casein. Additionally, the beta-casein in sheep and goat milk is the A2 variant, which is less inflammatory than the A1 variant found in most cow milk. Research links A1 beta-casein to autism, diabetes,

IBS, IBD, and other inflammatory conditions. Interestingly, the A2 beta-casein variant is not linked to these conditions—at least, not yet.

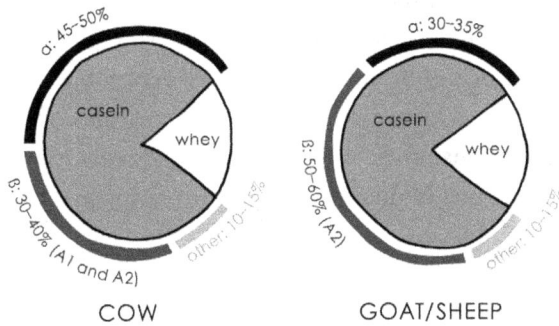

COW   GOAT/SHEEP

The casein in sheep and goat milk is smaller and more similar to human milk protein, making it easier to digest. However, casein is still casein. Beta-casein may be less inflammatory than alpha-casein, and A2 beta-casein may be less inflammatory than A1 beta-casein, but all casein can promote inflammation in an unhealthy gut.

Cross-reactivity is another issue. This phenomenon occurs when your immune system reacts to one form of casein (cow milk, for example) and develops antibodies against that protein. Exposure to a related protein (perhaps casein from goat or sheep milk) can activate the antibodies and trigger the immune system to mount a similar reaction. When the immune system fails to distinguish differences between two related proteins, cross-reactivity occurs. This reaction often occurs between A1 and A2 beta-casein. These proteins only differ by a single amino acid; therefore, if you have developed antibodies toward the A1 beta-casein common in cow milk, you may also experience the same symptoms when you consume A2 beta-casein. When this happens, goat or sheep milk no longer becomes a good substitute for cow milk.

The final issue with goat or sheep milk is the presence of lactose. Lactose is always counterproductive to gut healing, as we will learn next.

LACTOSE

Lactose is milk sugar and accounts for approximately 5 percent of milk content. It is responsible for milk's distinctive sweet taste. Lactose intolerance and maldigestion are extremely common problems, present in about 75 percent of all adults worldwide.[89] Infants produce small amounts of lactase, the enzyme that digests lactose, to efficiently assimilate their mother's milk. Once the baby begins to wean, though, lactase production diminishes. By the age of 5, most lactase production has ceased and lactose intolerance appears. Humans are the only creatures that continue the strange practice of consuming milk after being weaned, so it shouldn't be a surprise to discover our bodies rebelling against this practice.

In the small intestine, undigested lactose becomes a food source for bacteria and yeast. Gas, bloating, and abdominal pain are signs of lactose fermentation by the yeast and bacteria. Not only does this enable the growth of these organisms, provoking dysbiosis or SIBO, but the accumulating pressure stimulates intestinal movement, leading to the familiar episodes of diarrhea and abdominal pain, classic elements of IBS or IBD.

Fermentation is the only way to eliminate lactose from milk products. Therefore, unsweetened yogurt and kefir are safe options if lactose is your only concern with milk.

RAW DAIRY

Raw dairy is healthier than conventional because live enzymes are present to aid in its digestibility and heat-sensitive nutrients are still intact. Moreover, nonhomogenized raw milk will not contain the small fat particles associated with heart disease. But raw milk still contains casein, and this casein is still inflammatory. It also contains lactose.

WHEY PROTEIN

Whey protein comprises approximately 20 percent of the protein in milk. It is the main constituent of many commercial and pharmaceutical-grade protein powders because of its high-quality amino acid profile. Whey protein does not contain casein or lactose, eliminating the issues associated with either component. Whey protein from raw milk supplies immunoglobulins to boost the immune system, as well as the most ideal amino acids to repair villi. Protein is critical for healing the gut, and whey protein shakes are a convenient option for obtaining additional amino acids. In the next chapter, we will discuss how to choose the right kind of whey protein.

Those with a true dairy allergy should avoid whey since cross-reactivity can cause an allergic reaction to any component of dairy, including whey.

THE BOTTOM LINE FOR GUT HEALING

There are multiple problems with consuming dairy, regardless of its animal origin. Conventional dairy floods the gut with damaging hormones and antibiotics. Casein proteins trigger inflammation and leaky gut. Lactose sugars offer a fermentable feast to yeast and bacteria. For these reasons, I recommend avoiding dairy if your gut health is a priority to you.

ELIMINATE COMPLETELY

- All commercial dairy products
- All milk products, including organic, raw, etc.
  - Cheese
  - Yogurt
  - Ice cream
  - Cream or half-and-half
- All foods with dairy (dressings, crackers, spice mixes, condiments, etc.)

USE SPARINGLY

- Unsweetened kefir (contains casein)
- Butter from grass-fed cows, if tolerated (contains trace amounts of casein)
- Daiya cheese (dairy-, casein-, lactose-, gluten-, and soy-free, but highly processed and may be inflammatory for some people. Only use this as an occasional treat.)

SAFE DAIRY OPTIONS & ALTERNATIVES

- Ghee (clarified butter free of casein)

- Whey protein concentrates (if minimally processed and from raw milk of grass-fed cows)

- Unsweetened coconut, almond, hemp, or flax milk

- Full-fat, unsweetened, canned coconut milk or coconut cream

- Water or coconut kefir

- Unsweetened, plain coconut-based "yogurt"

Chapter Summary: Dairy causes many problems for the gut, making it a poor nutritional choice for healing. Casein is not easily digested and triggers an inflammatory reaction, which aggravates leaky gut. Lactose is sugar that feeds yeast and bad bacteria, contributing to dysbiosis. Commercial dairy contains residues of veterinary drugs, including antibiotics and hormones, which disrupt the gut microbiota and damage the villi. Goat and sheep milk, as well as raw, grass-fed cow milk, still contain casein and lactose, making them unhelpful for healing the gut.

CHAPTER 15:

MEAT AND PROTEIN

S O FAR, WE HAVE EXAMINED food groups that hinder gut healing. You may be wondering what food groups are safe to eat. In this chapter, we will introduce the safe food groups and learn how they help heal the gut, as well as how to make healthy food choices.

Proteins are integral for healing because they form the core of our physical structure. Proteins are the building blocks for our cells, enzymes, hormones, neurotransmitters, immune factors, and every other structure in the human body. Your entire body functions because of proteins.

Thousands of individual amino acids link together to create a 3D structure called protein. There are only 20 amino acids, but they can be arranged in thousands of sequences to create a myriad of different protein structures. Each structure has a unique 3D shape that determines its function in the body. Your DNA is like a book full of recipes and instructions for building these protein structures.

To understand how this process works in the body, let's look at an example. When you eat carbohydrates, your pancreas must produce the correct digestive enzyme, amylase, to break long starch molecules into single glucose molecules. The pancreas doesn't keep a supply of amylase handy. Instead, as carbohydrates enter your mouth, neurons deliver messages to the brain, alerting it to the presence of carbohydrates. The brain responds by sending signals to the cells of the pancreas telling them to make amylase. In a pancreas cell, special molecules search through the DNA's "recipes" to find instructions for making amylase. Once identified, the cell gathers the correct amino acids and arranges them according to the instructions in the DNA. Once assembled, the amino acid chain folds into the 3D protein structure for amylase. It's delivered to the small intestine and starts digesting the carbohydrates.

This same process is repeated to make hormones, antibodies, neurotransmitters, and the various components of our cells. When the need arises, the body gathers the recipes and instructions from the DNA, assembles the amino acids, and supplies the correct protein structure that will function as the necessary hormone, antibody, neurotransmitter, etc.

When you consume foods with protein, hydrochloric acid in the stomach unfolds the protein structures and disassembles the amino acids. The amino acids travel to the small intestine, where more enzymes (proteases) ensure their digestion into individual components is complete. The villi absorb the amino acids into the bloodstream, where they replenish the body's amino acid pool and remain stored until they are needed to make new proteins.

Are you beginning to understand why proteins are so important for healing? A broken body requires new structures and substances to repair the old. When infections and inflammation destroy the villi, the body must build new villi cells using amino acids. The chicken, fish, beef, beans, nuts, and seeds you eat supply the amino acids necessary to build these structures, as well as antibodies, hormones, enzymes, chemical messengers, and transporters. This process is an example of renewable energy sourcing at its best.

Let's now turn our attention to the healthiest options for replenishing our amino acid supply.

INDUSTRIALIZED MEATS

In the past 60 years, the growth of the fast-food industry has changed the face of our farms and the food they produce. Before this time, cows grazed on luscious green pastures, chickens pecked around the grounds of the farm, pigs scavenged in barnyards, and family units cared for these animals. The entrepreneurial idea of "meals on wheels" (roller skates, that is) soon morphed into a culture of fast food. The demand for uniform meat increased substantially, and the industrialization of farms was born. There simply wasn't enough time to allow cows to graze in fields, nor to allow chickens their full 90-day maturation period. After all, chicken nuggets and burgers were the new American classics. In addition to our changing palates, government subsidy programs such as the school lunch program, SNAP, and Meals on Wheels were growing at rapid rates, increasing the demand for more meat at a lower cost.

In response to these changes, large, industrial, concentrated animal feeding operations (CAFOs) began supplying the meat previously provided by family farms. Antibiotics and growth hormones shortened the maturation period for all meat animals. Breeding programs were implemented to genetically alter chickens toward larger-breasted birds to meet the demand for white meat. Grain-based diets fattened cattle and hastened their journey to the slaughterhouse. The stressful living conditions and slaughtering procedures elevated the stress hormones in the animals, which further increased their weight and weakened their immune systems, making them prone to diseases. The toxic ammonia gases rising from concentrated animal excrement restricts human exposure to these facilities. Ironically, the animals are forced to breathe these same toxic fumes their entire lives. The outcome of these changes was a steady supply of uniform beef, chicken, pork, eggs, and dairy.

What began as a sound economic move has become an environmental and health hazard. The close living quarters and sickly conditions of the animals have led to massive increases in bacterial outbreaks and unavoidable contamination of hundreds of pounds of meat. Antibiotic resistance and "superbugs" have become a medical threat as CAFOs have increased bacterial resistance to life-saving drugs. In response to this problem, new technology including irradiation[j] was developed to manage the rising levels of bacteria. Environmental contamination is a continual problem, since CAFOs produce thousands of gallons of polluted animal waste that are absorbed into our waterways, soil, and air.

We have sacrificed food quality in our desire to mass-produce food at a

---

j Treating food with ionizing radiation to kill bacteria and parasites.

lower cost. The inexpensive animal protein displayed in most of our grocery stores contains gut-destroying drugs and hormones, inflammatory fats, and infectious organisms. This food is not the same food that was produced by small family farms and consumed by mankind throughout history.

GRASS-FED MEATS

Quality is crucial when choosing healthy proteins to heal the body. To avoid the issues posed by drugs, hormones, inflammatory fats, bacteria, and toxic gases, we must choose to consume meat from animals raised in their natural environment with constant access to fresh pasture and clean air and water.

Grass-fed cows, lambs, and sheep contain many nutritional elements that grain-fed animals don't possess.

Grass-fed meat has less fat overall. The fat it does supply contains healthy, anti-inflammatory omega-3 fatty acids and conjugated linoleic acid (CLA). Research shows us the saturated fat found in grass-fed meat doesn't elevate cholesterol levels like inflammatory saturated fats from grain-fed meat.[90]

A diet of grass transfers several antioxidant nutrients such as vitamins A and E and glutathione (the chief antioxidant in the body) to the animal's meat and fat. These antioxidants neutralize the damaging free radicals generated by the toxins in our body. The drug and hormone residues found in conventionally raised meat increases these free radicals and exposes our liver to toxic drugs it will need to detoxify.

Health advocates have cautioned us against eating too much beef because of its role in inflammatory health conditions such as cardiovascular disease and cancer. Although all "red" meat contains some level of inflammatory saturated fats, grass-fed beef boasts lower levels of inflammatory saturated fats and balances them with anti-inflammatory omega-3 fats. Conventional beef not only contains high levels of inflammatory saturated fats but also lacks any anti-inflammatory fats, which are created when cattle eat grass.

FREE-RANGE/CAGE-FREE POULTRY & EGGS

Chickens raised in CAFO farms also experience bacterial infections, toxic fumes, and poor diets that render their meat less than healthy. The FDA finally restricted the use of hormones in poultry, but their feed still contains antibiotics, animal blood, diseased animal parts, litter waste, and genetically modified grains. The antibiotic residues found in poultry meat damage our gut microbiota just as when we take a course of antibiotics.

Researchers continue to investigate the potential health consequences of feeding animals genetically modified, grain-based diets. Animal studies show changes in intestinal cell structure and growth when they are fed a genetically modified diet. It is possible that the genetically modified organisms are transferred to humans when we consume animals fed these diets, and that they could cause similar changes in our gut. As our guts become less healthy and the incidence of chronic disease rises, we are prompted to investigate all agents that could be sabotaging our gut health, including genetically modified organisms.

The birds' living conditions present another health issue. Conventionally raised caged chickens spend their lives in cramped, dark cages that scarcely allow movement. They are often diseased, their bodies disabled, and many die. Dead chickens can remain caged with live chickens for several days, spreading disease. Humanely raised free-range birds have full access to pasture and engage in their natural behaviors of roaming, perching, and pecking at insects and plants. These birds are less stressed, less diseased, and less toxic.

Sadly, "cage-free" is now a trendy label for poultry products, and one with loose definitions. As food manufacturers scramble to capitalize on a population sector that demands humanely raised poultry products, they have adopted the "cage-free" label without properly disclosing the facts. The consumer may envision chickens roaming in the fresh outdoors, but a deeper investigation reveals windowless chicken houses sheltering thousands of chickens. They may not be in cages, but they don't have room to roam, nor access to the outdoors. The crowded, contaminated environment still subjects the birds to disease and toxins.

Food manufacturers also abuse the "free-range" label and apply it to conventional poultry houses that allow birds minimal room to roam and have limited windows for ventilation. This situation is still a far cry from the small family poultry farms that used to pepper the countryside.

"Certified Humane Raised and Handled®" is another label you may see on poultry. This nonprofit organization holds farmers to higher standards that allow poultry noncompetitive access to fresh water and food, an environment that encourages natural behaviors, and air quality that is comfortable for human exposure. Although this label still doesn't describe the environment of a small family farm, it may offer the best situation available among mass poultry producers.

Clearly, we must be careful with labels. Whenever possible, investigate the manufacturer. Cage-free poultry is better than conventional. Free-range is better than cage-free. Humanely raised is better than free-range. Purchasing poultry from your local farmer, where you can verify the bird's environment, is the best option.

The chicken's living environment and diet affect egg production and nutrition. The real evidence of a naturally raised chicken is in the egg. Does it have a hard shell? Is the yolk dark yellow or orange? Is the consistency of the egg white thick rather than runny? These are signs of an egg bursting with nutrition.

A nutritional comparison between the eggs of pastured, free-range hens and conventional USDA eggs showed that pastured eggs provided the following dietary benefits:[91]

- 1/3 less cholesterol
- 1/4 less saturated fat
- 2/3 more vitamin A
- 2 times more omega-3 fatty acids
- 3 times more vitamin E
- 7 times more beta carotene

A dark yellow or orange yoke reveals more vitamin A-derived antioxidants, such as lutein and zeaxanthin. A hard shell is indicative of high mineral content, and a thick egg white is a measure of freshness. Eggs from pastured chickens are less likely to carry dangerous diseases such as *Salmonella* and *E. coli*, which are prevalent in commercial eggs. With their additional healing nutrients and a lower risk of contamination, high-quality eggs offer an excellent source of protein.

FARMED VS. WILD-CAUGHT SEAFOOD

Fish and seafood are important protein sources for the gut. Unfortunately, many of us prefer a juicy red burger or grilled chicken over fresh fish and seafood. But as medical burdens rise, we are often forced to make wiser choices in our food selections. Fish and seafood contain more anti-inflammatory omega-3 fatty acids than any other food group. As a source of both anti-inflammatory fats and protein, fish becomes a gut-healing elixir.

We must be selective when choosing seafood for our health. Fish and seafood are also victims of modern food industrialization. Fish farms are the aquatic version of CAFOs. Large quantities of fish live in commercial holding tanks and consume a genetically modified, grain-based diet, laced with antibiotics to keep diseases at bay. Farmed fish live in water littered with their waste and treated with pesticides to combat sea lice. Toxin levels are substantial and commonly found in the flesh of farmed fish.[92]

Consequently, farmed fish don't acquire healthful anti-inflammatory omega-3 fatty acids without being supplemented with fish oil. Fish typically accrue omega-3 fats from a natural diet of seaweed and plankton. In the absence of these food sources, fish lack anti-inflammatory fats. Given that this is the primary reason we eat fish, farmed fish is no longer a sustainable protein source because its nutritional value is dependent on supplementation. Fish oil is increasingly harder for fisheries to obtain, forcing restrictions on the amount given to fish and resulting in a fish supply with steadily decreasing levels of omega-3 fatty acids.[93]

Additional problems arise because fisheries are supplementing with vegetable oils that increase pro-inflammatory omega-6 fatty acids. As the balance of omega-6 and omega-3 fats shifts toward the more inflammatory fats, fish is losing its status as a gut-healing elixir. This dilemma exacerbates a larger health problem as our dietary sources of pro-inflammatory omega-6 fats become more prevalent.

Seafood can contain high levels of mercury and toxic metals. Some consumers have been falsely led to believe farming protects fish (and the humans that consume them) from toxic mercury. Mercury levels accumulate in wild fish when they consume other fish that contain mercury. The most toxic fish are predatory species with long lifespans during which they consume many mercury-laden fish. Large fish that eat other large fish with long lifespans are more prone to higher mercury levels. Swordfish, shark, king mackerel, marlin, tilefish, and some forms of tuna have higher levels of mercury. Since mercury toxicity is an issue of fish size and lifespan, small wild-caught fish (such as herring, anchovies, sardines) or those with short lifespans (salmon) have negligible risks for mercury toxicity. These wild-caught fish are safe to consume and free from the genetically modified feed, toxic pesticides, and antibiotics that are present in farmed fish. See the resources in Part 4 for a list of seafood types with average mercury levels.

Finally, you should be aware of the new FDA-approved genetically engineered salmon. Despite ongoing lawsuits from concerned consumers, AquaBounty Technologies in Massachusetts continues to bring these "Frankenfish" out to market. Research has not consistently proven genetically engineered foods are safe for human consumption, and their effects most often target the gut.

Wild-caught salmon, herring, anchovies, and sardines are the healthiest seafood choices, owing to their low toxicity and high omega-3 content. A 3-ounce salmon fillet contains nearly 2,200mg of omega-3 fats, making it twice as potent as traditional fish oil capsules. Both protein and anti-inflammatory omega-3 fatty acids are vital for gut healing, as they decrease inflammation and rebuild villi. Sustainable, wild-caught fish and seafood is a necessary part of a healthy, healing diet.

BONE BROTH

Bone broth is foundational for gut restoration. The nutrients offered are exclusive to that elixir and target the gut to repair damaged cells and leaky junctions.

Bone broth is not consumed for its vitamin and mineral content, as many assume. In fact, the most comprehensive nutritional analysis on bone broth failed to show any significant amounts of vitamins and minerals.[94] Many theorize that bone broth must contain the minerals found in bone—namely, calcium, magnesium, and phosphorus—but alas, the studies don't prove it. The only method that enriched bone broth with minerals involved the addition of vegetables and fresh herbs, which increased potassium levels substantially.

The healing component of bone broth is its unique protein source. As skin, joints, and cartilage simmer for hours, they release collagen, the unique protein that forms these connective tissues. Collagen is a component of intestinal cells that can be destroyed by a leaky gut or inflammatory gut conditions such as IBS and IBD.[95] Resupplying the gut with collagen propels healing and restoration.

In the process of making bone broth, collagen is broken down into gelatin, a substance rich in healing amino acids like glycine, proline, arginine, and glutamine. Glutamine is the food of the small intestine and helps to rebuild the villi. Gelatin also inhibits the production of inflammatory factors, reducing their numbers in the gut.[96]

Instructions for making a rich, gut-healing bone broth are provided in Part 4 of this book. This broth should be a daily part of your health regime.

If you find yourself consistently unable to make bone broth, collagen protein is available as a powdered drink mix. It can be found alongside traditional whey-, pea-, and rice-based protein powders. Only choose a collagen powder that is sourced from grass-fed, pasture-raised cows. Hydrolyzed collagen peptides are the easiest to digest.

THE SOY CONTROVERSY

Soy has created a controversy among health advocates for decades, one for which there is no sound solution. Weighing the pros against the cons and being comfortable with your personal choice is important. Most advocates of soy cite Asian dietary practices and favorable health outcomes in their defense. Indeed, soy is common in Asian cuisines and Asians have a low rate of chronic health conditions and estrogen-related conditions such as breast cancer. Research affirms the consumption of soy for these positive outcomes, but while soy may offer some health benefits, there are an equal number of potential dangers. Soy quality has become a large piece of this puzzle that may provide more definitive answers.

First, let's review the potential benefits of soy. It is the most bioavailable plant-based protein. Protein bioavailability is a measurement of its digestibility and availability to the body. The score depends on the presence of all nine essential amino acids, which we must obtain from our diet because the body cannot manufacture them. A protein that contains all nine essential amino acids is a complete protein with a high bioavailability score. Animal proteins are complete, with a bioavailability score between 80 and 100 percent, meaning our body can digest and utilize 80 to 100 percent of the amino acids. Most plant-based proteins have a bioavailability score of between 60 and 80 percent because many are missing some essential amino acids. Soy is the only complete plant-based protein with a high bioavailability score. For this reason, soy has been a staple protein source for vegans and vegetarians.

Research indicates soy may be beneficial for postmenopausal women, reducing their risks of cardiovascular disease, osteoporosis, and breast cancer and helping to manage symptoms of menopause. These outcomes are due to soy's ability to mimic estrogen. These same benefits appear when women take estrogen replacements during menopause. Controversies still exist regarding the safety of estrogen replacement and the purported advantages of maintaining active estrogen receptors at a time in life when estrogen is naturally decreasing.

Many arguments against soy focus on its phytoestrogens—compounds that mimic estrogen by attaching to estrogen receptors on cells. Initially, researchers thought this action protected women's bodies from estrogen-stimulated cancers because soy blocked estrogen's activity, but others claim it increases estrogenic activity because soy mimics estrogen's activity. Exposure to estrogen-mimicking toxins is growing through the use of plastics, chemicals in skin care products, and environmental contamination. Likewise, estrogen dominance is a legitimate problem among women, leading to reproductive issues and cancer. Many people question whether soy is contributing to this problem. Additionally, phytoestrogens in soy may compromise male fertility and act as endocrine (hormone) disruptors with a cascade of associated health conditions.[97] Soy-based infant formula is also highly controversial, as studies have shown that infants fed soy-based formula have phytoestrogen levels that surpass the normal estrogen levels of an adult woman.

So why do Asian cultures have lower incidences of estrogen-driven health conditions, despite their frequent soy consumption? The answer may be summed up in one word: quality. Soy in Asia hasn't been genetically modified, washed in toxic chemicals, and heavily processed into soy protein isolates (SPIs). But this modified form of soy dominates the American food supply, being present in nearly 80 percent of all processed foods. SPIs are used to make soy milk, soy-based infant formula, soy protein bars, soy cheese, soy-based meat alternatives, and other soy-based food products. Textured soy product, a processed form of genetically modified soy, is used by schools to fortify the food in the school lunch program. Processed, genetically modified soy is the prevailing form of soy in America.

In contrast, Asians consume soy in its unprocessed, non-genetically modified form. Tempeh, natto, and miso are fermented forms of unprocessed soy quite common in Asian cuisine. Tofu is not fermented, but is another non-processed, non-genetically modified form of whole soybeans.

If you choose to consume soy, I recommend organic, unaltered and, ideally, fermented soy. Soy protein isolates and other processed forms of soy are potentially detrimental to your health.

WHEY PROTEIN CONCENTRATES (NOT ISOLATES)

Whey protein can offer a litany of gut-healing benefits. It increases the growth of healthy bacteria, *Bifidobacterium* and *Lactobacillus,* while decreasing the number of harmful bacteria.[98] People with dysbiosis and SIBO can obviously benefit from this effect.

The immune-boosting properties of whey are impressive. It contains immunoglobulins (antibodies), the same critical immune boosters found in the colostrum of breast milk. Whey protein also improves the gut mucosal barrier and tightens the junctions between the cells, meaning it helps correct leaky gut.[99, 100] Whey protein can be a convenient and healthy source of gut-healing proteins, but as with everything, quality is key. The components that improve the immune system, gut barrier, and leaky cell junctions are only present in minimally processed whey protein concentrates sourced from exclusively grass-fed cows. It is best if the proteins are not denatured (disrupted by heat or acidity), as is the case in whey protein isolate, a not-so-healthy cousin to whey protein concentrate.

VEGANISM

Following a strict vegan nutritional plan while attempting to heal the gut is difficult. Vegan diets, by nature, rely on lots of carbohydrates. They don't have to include grains, but beans, legumes, nuts, and seeds are essential for obtaining adequate protein. Many of these plant-based protein sources are problematic for individuals with dysbiosis, leaky gut, and especially SIBO. As we have learned, the bacteria associated with dysbiosis and SIBO ferment these carbohydrates, producing large amounts of gas and pressure. Bloating, fullness, abdominal distention, pain, and other gut symptoms can become severe. Many individuals with SIBO temporarily eliminate these forms of carbohydrates to manage symptoms while rebalancing the gut microbiota. Unfortunately, removing these foods will make it virtually impossible for a vegan to obtain adequate protein for gut healing.

It is outside of the scope of this book to compare the health benefits of a vegan versus a paleo style of eating. A vast majority of the population finds a paleo style of eating (high protein, lower carb) is more powerful for restoring gut health compared to a vegan style of eating. And yet some people still derive significant health benefits from a vegan diet, giving evidence to our unique and individual requirements. The new and blossoming field of nutrigenomics[k] may shed more light on this issue in the future. It is not my desire to sway your attitude or belief regarding either of these dietary preferences. Both have been powerful tools for restoring health and vitality.

---

k   The study of the interaction between nutrition and genetics and how it may prevent disease.

Rather, this book focuses on the nutritional plan that will benefit most of its readers.

THE BOTTOM LINE FOR GUT HEALING

Protein is one of the most important nutrients for healing the gut. It supplies critical amino acids to repair villi, rebuild barriers, tighten the loose junctions of leaky gut, and restore the integrity of the gut. Meanwhile, it helps starve yeast and harmful bacteria while satisfying your appetite. Unfortunately, the industrialization of meat production complicates the issue. To obtain the healing benefits offered by this food group, you must make healthy, educated choices when purchasing meat and animal products.

Industrialization has also changed food economics. It is nearly impossible to turn a blind eye to the higher costs and relative scarcity of well-sourced, pastured protein. Quality is more important in this food group than any other. At the very least, it is imperative that you purchase hormone-free, antibiotic-free meat, poultry, and eggs. Antibiotic and hormone residues encourage dysbiosis, inflammation, and gut destruction. If you are able to obtain it, organic is a good option, but grass-fed, pastured meats and poultry from a local farmer are your best choices. Wild-caught fish should be consumed weekly for its anti-inflammatory fats. Bone broth should be a routine part of any gut-healing diet.

ELIMINATE COMPLETELY

- Conventional beef or pork
- Conventional poultry and eggs
- Farm-raised fish and seafood
- Soy protein isolates/textured soy protein
- Swordfish, shark, king mackerel, tilefish, albacore tuna, orange roughy, grouper, halibut

USE OCCASIONALLY
(up to once a week)

- Humanely raised, pastured pork

- Organic, non-fermented soy (tofu)
- Sustainable, wild-caught light tuna, shellfish, haddock, pollock, flounder, trout, catfish

SAFE PROTEIN

- Bone broth
- Grass-fed, pastured beef
- Humanely raised, free-range poultry and eggs
- Sustainable, wild-caught salmon, herring, anchovies, sardines, tilapia
- Minimally processed whey protein concentrates, sourced from grass-fed cattle
- Hydrolyzed collagen peptides, sourced from grass-fed, pastured animals
- Fermented soy (natto, tempeh, miso), for vegans or vegetarians

Chapter Summary: Proteins supply the body with amino acids, the building blocks for every cell, molecule, and substance in the body. Animal products offer the most bioavailable protein. Grass-fed beef, free-range poultry and eggs, and wild-caught fish are the healthiest choices. Bone broth and collagen protein are gut-healing elixirs. If you choose soy, only consume organic (non-GMO), fermented whole soy. Significant controversy overshadows any potential benefit of soy, so investigate the issues before you decide to consume this protein. Minimally processed whey protein concentrate from grass-fed cattle is a convenient protein option with many additional gut-healing benefits.

CHAPTER 16:

VEGETABLES AND FRUITS

VEGETABLES AND FRUITS: HERE LIES the cornerstone of all nourishing diets. Whether vegan or paleo, healing or healthy, vegetables and fruits are vital sources of all vitamins, minerals, antioxidants, and phytonutrients. No dietary plan or nutritional philosophy dares to argue with the essential nature of this food group. Let the nutritional debates swirl around grains, proteins, and fats, but as for this food group, give me plenty, or give me death.

In our industrialized world where sugar, fat, and salt have reprogrammed our tongue's preference for authentic flavors, vegetables have become the bad kid sitting in the corner of the plate. Fruit, being naturally sweet, still holds an acceptable position among even the pickiest eater, but it can be quickly passed over for ice cream. Vegetables and fruit offer the greatest variety, creativity, flavor, and color of any food group, but in our nutritional stupor, we have replaced beautiful bounty with mysterious mush.

A RAINBOW OF COLORS

The broad color scheme of the vegetable and fruit families expresses the variety of vitamins, minerals, antioxidants, and phytonutrients they contain. Each color represents a distinct nutritional profile.

- **Red** reveals vitamin A and its derivatives (carotenoids and retinol), as well as the antioxidants lycopene, lutein, and zeaxanthin. These nutrients nourish the skin and eyes.

- **Purple and blue** pigmentation indicates the antioxidant anthocyanin, which protects against cancer, cardiovascular disease, and stroke.

- **Dark green** contains many phytonutrients, including indoles and saponins that protect against cancer.

- **White** vegetables often contain allicin, which acts as an antimicrobial agent.

Each color group targets different areas of the body, making it vital to include every color of vegetable in our diets if we are going to experience whole-body health.

ANTIOXIDANTS

Vegetables and fruit deliver more antioxidants than any other food group. These nutrients are more vital today for maintaining health than at any other time in history. Why? Because we are bombarded with toxic substances that produce free radicals at an overwhelming rate. Antioxidants act as our body's housekeepers. They scour the body for damaging free radicals with the mission to kill them before they weaken and destroy our body.

Free radicals play a primary role in the progression of nearly every known health condition. Sometimes they may initiate the disease process, such as with cancer, but other times, the disease process generates free radicals and they become responsible for the progressive nature of the disease. Diabetes is an example of this phenomenon. High blood sugar produces free radicals, which can damage the neurological system, kidneys, and other organs, explaining the degenerative nature of diabetes.

The body generates free radicals to engage an infectious agent or toxin in battle. It intends for the free radicals to kill the infectious organism or toxin. With the job completed, antioxidants move in to clean up the free radicals before they attack healthy cells.

Other mechanisms that generate free radicals in our body include:

- Electromagnetic fields from cell phones, the electrical grid, radioactive waves, and radiological medical procedures such as X-rays, MRI scans, and ultrasounds

- Toxic products of cigarette smoke, environmental pollution, and household chemicals
- Unhealthy foods, preservatives, additives, and excessive sugar
- Extreme exercise and long cardiovascular exercise events
- Chronic stress

It is nearly impossible to escape all the destructive forces that burden our bodies with free radicals, but we can equip ourselves with a host of antioxidants by consuming more vegetables and fruits.

An unhealthy gut can contain massive amounts of free radicals because of infections, toxins, unhealthy foods, and inflammation. Once generated, the damaging molecules begin destroying intestinal cells. Controlling free radicals is not only important for our entire body, but is also crucial if we are going to heal our gut.

ALKALINIZING POWER

The healing power of vegetables and fruits is not only present in their rich supply of vitamins, minerals, antioxidants, and phytonutrients; they also keep our body's pH alkaline. There has been renewed interest in the acid/alkaline element of healing, and for a good reason! Many disease processes gain momentum in an acidic environment. Every cancer cell creates an acid "bubble" around itself so it can survive and reproduce more efficiently. Demolishing this acid bubble is one means of lowering cancer's survival rate.

A diet of processed grains, sugar, and commercial meat and dairy establishes an acidic environment in the body. As the blood struggles to maintain the neutral pH required for life, it pulls calcium and magnesium from the body's storehouse to buffer the excess acid. Where are calcium and magnesium stored? In our bones. An acid diet can cause osteoporosis, despite adequate consumption of calcium-rich foods. To preserve our calcium supplies, we must offer the body alkalinizing foods such as vegetables and fruit.

It is important to realize that a high-protein diet will produce a highly acidic environment unless we balance it with a plethora of alkalinizing vegetables and fruits. A good rule of thumb is to make sure 20 percent of your diet comes from quality proteins and healthy fats, while the remaining 80 percent should focus on nutrient-rich, alkalinizing vegetables and fruits so that you can maintain a healthy, healing pH.

HEALTHY CARBOHYDRATES

Vegetables and fruits should supply most of the carbohydrates our bodies need to function. They are a carbohydrate powerhouse because this food group not only provides carbohydrates, but delivers them along with fiber to help sustain a healthy blood sugar. These carbohydrates also include vitamins, minerals, and phytonutrients to help the body metabolize glucose efficiently.

Each vegetable or fruit possesses a different amount of carbohydrates, allowing for variability based on our needs. For example, white potatoes contain a significant amount of starch and comparatively little fiber and nutrients. After eating white potatoes, the body quickly digests the starch into glucose. This glucose feeds yeast and bacteria in the gut. It also causes a temporary spike in your blood sugar. Dark leafy greens furnish lots of alkalinizing vitamins, minerals, and phytonutrients while supplying very few carbohydrates. The unique nutrient profile of vegetables allows them to complement each other in the body. For this reason, it is important to consume a variety of vegetables and fruit.

If you recall, bacteria and yeast feast on high-starch carbohydrates, so while we work on rebalancing our gut microbiome, it is necessary to identify and avoid starchy vegetables and fruits, at least temporarily.

The glycemic load (GL) is a helpful tool for measuring the starch in vegetables and fruits. It indicates how many carbohydrates are delivered in a serving of food. It also considers the speed at which the body digests starch into glucose. When starving the yeast and harmful bacteria in your gut, it is important to choose low-GL vegetables and fruits. All your most frequently consumed foods should have a GL of less than 10, but the lower the GL, the easier it is to starve out the infections and heal the gut. In Part 4, you will find a recommended website to help you discover the GL for many types of foods.

FRUIT AND SUGAR

Unquestionably, fruit is a nutrient-rich, alkalinizing, antioxidant powerhouse and should be part of any healthy diet. Nevertheless, the bacteria and yeast in an unhealthy gut consume the naturally occurring sugars in fruit and use them to survive and reproduce. When dysbiosis is present, the organisms send messages to the brain when they are hungry, and the brain then signals a craving for sugar, carbohydrates, and fruit.

The naturally occurring sugars in fruit are certainly healthier than refined, processed sugar. Fruit sugar is bound to fiber that slows its digestion and absorption. Fruit also contains a unique prebiotic fiber that feeds the beneficial bacteria (probiotics) in the gut. This design is incredible because fruit sugar (also known as fructose) creates a lot of distress in the intestine when it is not bound to fiber, because the intestinal cells don't readily absorb fructose. Instead, fiber presents fructose to the cells at a rate they can accommodate.

Unfortunately, an unbalanced microbiota can misinterpret the benefits of fruit and starchy vegetables. As bacteria and yeast feed on the sugars and starch, they produce gaseous byproducts that cause bloating, gas, and abdominal distention and pain. While the gut is healing, only low-sugar fruits and low-starch vegetables are beneficial for rebalancing the microbiota.

SIBO, IBS, AND FODMAPs

Vegetables and fruit are healthy sources of carbohydrates, but people struggling with certain gut conditions must be selective regarding their choices in this food group.

The bacteria associated with SIBO (small intestinal bacterial overgrowth) and IBS (irritable bowel syndrome) are notorious for causing unpleasant symptoms in the presence of certain healthy carbohydrates. Remember, SIBO occurs when the normal, healthy bacteria of the colon overgrow and spill over into the small intestine. In their normal environment, the bacteria feed on fiber without causing any problems. In the small intestine, the gaseous byproducts of fermenting fiber cause bloating and abdominal distention and pain.

Many IBS patients suffer from SIBO. As the gaseous byproducts of fermentation increase the pressure in the small intestine, it triggers symptoms of IBS.

Both SIBO and IBS show clinical improvement when the diet is devoid of specific groups of fermentable carbohydrates, identified by the acronym FODMAP.[101] FODMAPs include:

- **F**ermentable

- **O**ligosaccharides: onions, garlic, legumes, chicory, artichokes, inulin, many grains, lentils

- **D**isaccharides: dairy products

- **M**onosaccharides: fructose such as honey, apples, pears, mango, watermelon

- **A**nd

- **P**olyols: sorbitol, mannitol, maltitol, xylitol, avocado, apples, apricots, nectarines, plums

Many vegetables and fruits contain FODMAPs. If you suffer from SIBO or IBS, you will need to eliminate these otherwise healthful foods while rebalancing the gut microbiota. Many online resources will help you identify foods that contain FODMAPs, but a comprehensive review of these foods is outside the scope of this book.

MORE VEGETABLES, LESS FRUITS

I would be remiss if I left you with the idea that vegetables and fruits occupy equal roles in a healthy diet. Although our taste buds may prefer sweet fruits, the body requires a heavy dose of vegetables for healing. Fruit contains natural sugars that feed yeast and bacteria, and therefore, we must consume them sparingly while we heal the gut. Remember, the first "R" of the "4R" plan is to *remove* foods that feed infectious organisms. Our goal is to starve and kill the organisms. The types of fruit we choose for a gut-healing diet should be low-sugar, high-antioxidant options.

MOLD

The last issue we must address is mold. Mold is counterproductive to gut healing because it triggers a strong immune response and inflammation. Research tells us mold (both environmental and dietary) has the power to comprehensively destroy our health. Though significant, a complete review of this subject is beyond the scope of this book.

Healing the gut requires us to avoid all moldy foods. Both mold and *Candida* are fungi. The immune system can confuse them because they originate from the same lineage. This phenomenon is called cross-reactivity. If the immune system encounters food-borne mold, the antibodies previously created by a *Candida* infection can mistake mold as an enemy and mount an immune response. This reaction is detrimental to gut healing because an active immune system damages intestinal cells.

Berries and melons are notorious for harboring mold, unless they are local, in season, and freshly harvested or frozen. Most travel thousands of miles to reach the supermarket, during which time mold spores can reproduce in the dark, moist environment. Mushrooms, though usually sold as a vegetable, are really a mold—a fungus, that is. Almost all corn (technically a grain, but often confused with vegetables) contains *Aspergillus* spores. Dried fruit is both a high-sugar and a high-mold food. Of course, any overly ripe vegetable or fruit can harbor mold.

THE BOTTOM LINE FOR GUT HEALING

Vegetables and fruit should occupy the greatest amount of space on the plate for a gut-healing meal. They are the storehouses of vitamins, minerals, antioxidants, and phytonutrients, and are the major alkalinizing agents of our diet. Their beneficial effects are indisputable and they are not optional if we desire optimum health.

While working toward a healthier gut, we may have to temporarily eliminate certain high-starch vegetables that lack adequate fiber, high-sugar fruits, and moldy foods. Despite these limitations, I think you will find the large variety of remaining options leaves much room for culinary creativity.

ELIMINATE COMPLETELY

- FODMAPs, if SIBO or IBS is a problem (see Resources for FODMAP lists)
- Moldy vegetables or fruits
- White potatoes
- Corn
- Out-of-season berries or melons
- Dried fruit
- Canned or processed fruit
- Fruit juices

USE SPARINGLY
(Only fresh or frozen, in small quantities, 1 to 2 times each week, with a protein-rich meal)

- Sweet potatoes (should be eliminated in advanced gut conditions)
- Beets
- Parsnips
- Pineapple
- Banana
- Mango
- Grapes
- Papaya

SAFE VEGETABLES AND FRUITS
(Only fresh or frozen; no canned or processed varieties)

- All vegetables not otherwise listed above
- Grapefruit
- Berries (only local, seasonally fresh or frozen)
- Citrus fruit (lemons, limes, oranges)

- Cherries

- Peaches

- All other fruit not listed above can be consumed in small quantities only

Note: Safe vegetables and fruits should have a GL of 6 or less. Vegetables and fruits with a GL between 10 and 15 should not be consumed more than once each week. A complete guide of GL measurements can be found under the Resources in this book.

Chapter Summary: Vegetables and fruit are rich in vitamins, minerals, antioxidants, and phytonutrients. Each color group represents a different nutrient profile. They alkalinize the body, creating a hostile environment for diseases. A healthful diet will include an abundance and variety of vegetables and fruit to replace the grain-based carbohydrates that do not promote healing. When healing the gut, we must avoid high-starch vegetables, high-sugar fruits, and foods that harbor mold.

CHAPTER 17:
BEANS AND LEGUMES

B EANS AND LEGUMES (INCLUDING LENTILS and peas) act as a double-edged sword in gut health. On the one hand, they serve as an important food source for the beneficial bacteria in the gut and therefore help to maintain the colonies. On the other hand, beans and legumes contain copious amounts of starch that can be fermented by yeast and bacteria, creating gaseous byproducts that trigger bloating, abdominal distention, and pain.

ANTI-NUTRIENTS

Another concern regarding beans and legumes is that they contain unhealthy anti-nutrients such as lectins, enzymes inhibitors, and phytates. These bind up certain vitamins, minerals, and nutrients and prevent their digestion and absorption. Lectins (as we noted with grains) can damage intestinal cells, leading to inflammation and a leaky gut.[102] Phytates (or phytic acid) can bind zinc, iron, and other minerals, rendering them unavailable to the body and diminishing the nutritional quality of the food. Phytates can inhibit enzymes required to break down proteins and starch. Individuals with an unhealthy, damaged gut already have problems with poor digestion, and phytates complicate the situation. Beans and legumes aren't the only foods that contain high levels of phytates. Spinach, swiss chard, nuts, seeds, and cacao also have phytates.

HEALTH BENEFITS

Beans and legumes provide an excellent source of food (i.e., fiber) for beneficial bacteria. They also offer a source of potassium, magnesium, folate, iron, zinc, antioxidants, and an impressive amount of amino acids. Beans and legumes are a rare plant-based source of the amino acid lysine, which makes them a vital part of a vegan diet.

Both fiber and lectins bind the glucose molecules produced from digested starch. This action prevents a quick spike in blood sugar by preventing the absorption of glucose. Instead, bound glucose slowly absorbs through the villi, which is helpful for maintaining a healthy blood sugar level, especially for people with diabetes.[103] By regulating blood sugar and increasing satiety, fiber aids in weight loss.[104] Finally, fiber, potassium, and the blood sugar-regulating effects of beans and legumes can reduce blood pressure and guard against heart disease.[105] Certainly, beans and legumes confer some significant health benefits.

SOAKING, COOKING, FERMENTING, AND SPROUTING

With all the positive elements of beans and legumes, it seems a shame to eliminate them from the diet. Thankfully, if we prepare beans and legumes correctly, we can potentially eliminate the vast majority of their unfavorable components.

Soaking beans and legumes for 12 to 24 hours before cooking them pre-digests some of the starch (oligosaccharides) responsible for producing excess gas and intestinal distress. Soaking reduces the phytate concentration by 20 to 30 percent and thus enhances nutrient availability.[106]

Both phytates and lectins are resistant to heat, but lectins are moderately neutralized by cooking. The higher the heat or pressure you apply during the cooking process, the more neutralization of lectins occurs. If pressure cooking is possible, this is the best solution. Phytates, on the other hand, aren't reduced by cooking. This makes soaking prior to cooking an important step.

Fermentation can reduce phytates by up to 98 percent.[107] Once the phytate is removed, the minerals in beans and legumes are readily available to the body. During fermentation, naturally occurring microbes adjust the pH of the environment and use enzymes to break down phytates. Furthermore, the bacteria release organic acids that impart various health benefits and enhance the body's ability to absorb minerals.

Sprouting is another preparation method that increases the nutritional value of beans and legumes. Sprouting (or germination) reduces problematic starches and pre-digests protein to enhance the availability of the amino acids. Some antioxidant and phytonutrient levels increase during sprouting. Overall, sprouting boosts the nutritional components of beans and legumes by increasing their bioavailability to the body.[108]

THE BOTTOM LINE FOR GUT HEALING

Beans and legumes may present problems for some individuals, but can be part of a healthy diet for others. They offer some health benefits, but can also exacerbate gut conditions if your gut is not functioning optimally. Therefore, we can't apply a one-size-fits-all approach to this food group.

If you are attempting to eliminate FODMAPs due to SIBO or IBS, you must temporarily remove beans and legumes to prevent unpleasant effects and encourage healing. Likewise, if you have dysbiosis or leaky gut and experience gas and bloating after eating beans and legumes, you should probably eliminate them while your gut is healing.

There isn't any reason to avoid beans and legumes if you don't experience noticeable side effects after consuming them. They are an excellent source of fiber and help maintain a healthy population of bacteria in the gut. They should be properly prepared to maximize their health benefits. Soaking and cooking beans will neutralize most of the lectins. Sprouting and fermenting is an even better option to maximize the nutritional value while minimizing the anti-nutrients.

ELIMINATE COMPLETELY

- All beans and legumes, if you experience bloating, gas, abdominal distention, or pain after consuming them
- All canned beans and legumes with additives such as sugars and preservatives

USE SPARINGLY

- Cooked beans and legumes that have not been soaked, sprouted, or fermented

SAFE BEANS AND LEGUMES

- All soaked and cooked beans and legumes, but ideally those that have also been fermented or sprouted

Chapter Summary: Beans and legumes can be an excellent source of vitamins, minerals, fiber and protein, but anti-nutrients such as lectins and phytates can limit the availability of these nutrients. Soaking, cooking, fermenting and sprouting beans and legumes will decrease anti-nutrients and increase the availability of their nutritional components. The fiber in beans and legumes promotes the growth of beneficial bacteria in the gut, regulates blood sugar, aids in weight loss, and lowers blood pressure. The fiber and additional starch components can exacerbate SIBO and IBS symptoms and are problematic in those with a damaged gut. These individuals may have to eliminate beans and legumes temporarily.

CHAPTER 18:

NUTS AND SEEDS

Nuts and seeds are important sources of calories, healthy fats, and protein. They're one of the few food groups that contain abundant quantities of the antioxidant nutrient vitamin E. Other vitamins and minerals found in nuts and seeds include folate, calcium, magnesium, phosphorus, and potassium.[109] They have a high satiety value and provide a convenient snack option. Their "flours" can be useful in creating healthy, gut-healing treats.

What is the difference between nuts and seeds? Nuts are a plant's fruit, which is encased in a hard shell and contains one or more seeds. Often, we remove the hard shell before eating the fruit and seeds within. Examples include acorns, chestnuts, and hazelnuts.

Seeds are the propagative part of the plant (the embryo) and contain all the nutrients and elements necessary for new plant growth. Think of a seed as a fertilized egg that has not yet begun to grow. Examples of seeds include sesame seeds, poppy seeds, Brazil nuts, and pine nuts. As you can see, the suffix doesn't define the food group.

There is a third category known as drupes. Almonds, cashews, pecans, pistachios, coconuts, pecans, and walnuts are examples of drupes. A drupe is a soft seed encased in a hard shell and found in the middle of a fleshy fruit. We remove the fruit and shell before consuming the drupe. Sometimes we consume the fruit, but leave the shell and enclosed seed, such as when we eat dates, plums, and peaches, which are also drupes.

The nutritional content of nuts and seeds are similar except that seeds contain more fiber and B vitamins. Some seeds supply unique fatty acids, or nutrients not found in other nuts and seeds. For example, chia seeds are especially rich in omega-3 fatty acids, while Brazil nuts are one of the few rich sources of selenium.

We often mistake peanuts as nuts. Despite the name, they are legumes, identified by a pod containing many fruits (the peanuts). Other examples of legumes include peas, carob, and all beans.

RAW OR ROASTED, ORGANIC OR NOT

Raw, organic nuts and seeds are the best options to consume regularly. Nuts can fall prey to irradiation,[1] pasteurization, bleaching, dyes, and chemical soaks. Growers treat some varieties of nuts with pesticides and antifungals as well.

Roasting is not particularly harmful, especially if dry roasting is used, but two potential issues exist. First, many nuts and seeds are roasted in rancid, processed, genetically modified oils such as canola or cottonseed oil. These oils not only impart the dangers associated with genetically modified foods, but rancid, processed oils are highly inflammatory. Second, roasting can destroy fragile nutrients and antioxidants including vitamin E and may decrease the bioavailability of some fats and proteins.

On the other hand, dry roasting has some benefits. It can destroy some of the phytates contained in nuts and seeds. Remember, these anti-nutrients are present in many grains, beans, and legumes and they bind minerals, preventing your body from absorbing them. As with beans and legumes, soaking, sprouting, dehydrating, or roasting helps eliminate some phytates from nuts and seeds.

ALLERGIES & INFLAMMATION

There are some legitimate concerns with nuts and seeds related to gut healing. Like other food groups, we must consider individual circumstances when determining whether nuts and seeds are a good food choice for you.

---

1   Ionizing radiation to preserve food and stop microbial growth

If you have an allergy to tree nuts or peanuts, it is obviously best to avoid these. However, an authentic allergy to nuts is rare and exists primarily in children. Remember that leaky gut can initiate several food intolerances as the immune system reacts to undigested food particles entering the bloodstream. Nuts and seeds can present the same challenge as grains, beans, and legumes in those with leaky gut. In these cases, eliminating them until the gut begins to heal is a good idea. However, if you don't notice symptoms after consuming nuts, it is unnecessary to avoid them.

Similarly, those with IBS or SIBO who notice improvement in their symptoms when avoiding FODMAPs may have to avoid this food group temporarily. Like beans and legumes, nuts and seeds contain fiber that feeds healthy bacteria. Although beneficial for a healthy gut, the fermentation (eating) of fiber by bacteria can cause bloating, abdominal distension, and pain when the body's beneficial bacteria have crept into the small intestine, as occurs in SIBO. Again, individuality governs the decision to partake in nuts and seeds when SIBO or IBS exists.

Others have challenged the healthfulness of nuts and seeds based on their high content of polyunsaturated omega-6 fatty acids. Although this is a healthy fat, the balance between omega-6 and omega-3 fats can determine whether our body efficiently produces inflammatory factors. Consuming too many omega-6 fats encourages inflammation, whereas omega-3 fats restrain inflammation. The omega-6 fat content in nuts and seeds should not pose a problem if your diet includes a healthy dose of omega-3 fats from fish and seafood. Some nuts and seeds such as chia seeds, walnuts, and pecans contain compounds that become omega-3 fats, but these are not good sources of this anti-inflammatory fat.

The consensus in the scientific literature is that nuts and seeds are positive contributors to an anti-inflammatory diet. Studies have shown reduced inflammatory markers in those who consume nuts and seeds versus those who do not.[110]

A FUNGUS AMONG US

The presence of toxic mold spores and fungus on nuts and seeds presents a legitimate health concern, especially when *Candida* is present. For this reason, people attempting to heal their gut should avoid some varieties of nuts and seeds. Bulk nuts and seeds are susceptible to carrying mold spores, which can trigger an inflammatory response and divert the immune system away from healing. As we learned with *Candida*, a fungus, mold spores can permeate nearly every body tissue and elude the immune system.

Mycotoxins are toxic compounds released by mold and fungi. One particular fungus, *Aspergillus*, is notorious for producing the toxic and carcinogenic mycotoxin known as aflatoxin. Since peanuts grow in the moist ground, all are contaminated with *Aspergillus* and transfer some amount of aflatoxin to the consumer. When stored in large bins, the mold grows exponentially. Upon entering our country, all peanuts and peanut products are tested for aflatoxin and must fall below a specified limit before being sold.[111] The unfortunate reality is that peanuts and peanut butter are staple food items in many households, and it's impossible to quantify how much of this toxin enters our systems. Government policy may establish acceptable levels, but the cumulative intake can easily surpass this limit. The unknown toxin load makes peanuts a great concern for our general health, and especially for those attempting to heal their gut.

Unfortunately, mold and fungi are detected on almost all types of nuts and seeds.[112, 113] The question is rarely *whether* mold exists, but rather, how much exists. The levels are dependent on storage techniques. In extremely mold-sensitive individuals, eliminating all nuts and seeds may be necessary. It is counterintuitive to introduce any mold into the diet, but the reality is that many foods, including fruits and vegetables, contain some amount of mold. Most individuals can tolerate the varieties of nuts and seeds that have lower mold counts and are sourced from locations or companies that minimize the likelihood of mold growth.

THE BOTTOM LINE FOR GUT HEALING

Nuts and seeds offer an excellent source of nutrients and calories that can impart many health benefits and provide variety as part of a healthy diet. They also supply an alternative source of protein, anti-inflammatory fats, and some antioxidant nutrients, all of which can benefit the gut. Nuts and seeds can be a problem if you have a nut allergy, SIBO, or IBS. In the latter cases, temporary elimination may be necessary, with the goal of reintroducing this food group after healing has progressed and tolerance has been re-established. It is important to choose organic and raw nuts and seeds to reduce toxin exposure and ensure the most nutrition. Purchase only fresh, regionally sourced nuts and seeds to reduce mold contamination, which can hinder gut healing and activate the immune system. Finally, peanuts (a legume) should be avoided altogether due to their contamination by toxic mold compounds, which undoubtedly impedes healing.

ELIMINATE COMPLETELY

- All nuts and seeds with sweet, sugary, or other coatings
- All nuts and seeds roasted in canola, cottonseed, safflower, soybean, or vegetable oil
- Peanuts, peanut butter, and peanut products

USE SPARINGLY

- Raw pistachios, cashews, and Brazil nuts, due to higher mold counts
- Non-organic nuts and seeds
- Nuts or seeds roasted in non-GMO oils

SAFE NUTS & SEEDS

- Raw, dry-roasted, or dehydrated nuts and seeds sourced from the US
- Nut and seed butters that don't contain added ingredients other than salt

Chapter Summary: Nuts and seeds are good sources of protein, healthy fats, fiber, vitamins, and minerals. Nuts can fall prey to irradiation, pasteurization, bleaching, dyes, chemical soaks, and roasting in genetically modified oils. Therefore, safer choices include organic, raw, dehydrated, or dry-roasted options. Those with nut allergies, SIBO, or IBS should avoid all nuts and seeds. Since all nuts and seeds contain mold, you should only consume low-mold varieties. You should avoid all peanuts, which contain high levels of toxic mold.

CHAPTER 19:

OILS AND FATS

F ALSE INFORMATION REGARDING FATS HAS caused a great deal of fear and confusion. With so many fat-alternative options available, who wouldn't be overwhelmed? As manufacturing companies compete to stake their claim in the marketplace, more convenient and inexpensive products emerge. Overwhelmed consumers decide to either abandon fats altogether and avoid the potential for harm, or casually purchase the most popular product, throwing all caution to the wind.

The problem with all this is that our bodies require certain fats to survive. Fat is required for every cell in our body to maintain its structure and function. Fat is necessary for building hormones and utilizing the fat-soluble vitamins (D, A, K, and E). The inflammatory response is directly impacted by fats in our diet. It isn't a surprise that fats play an essential role in healing the gut.

To remove some of the mystery surrounding fats, we must first discuss the different forms of fat.

TYPES OF FATS

Fats fall into two broad categories: saturated and unsaturated. They can be identified by the fact that saturated fats are solid at room temperature, while unsaturated fats are liquid.

Unsaturated fats are further divided into polyunsaturated (including omega-3 and omega-6 fatty acids) and monounsaturated (including omega-9 fatty acids) fats.

SATURATED FATS

Saturated fats are widely misunderstood and most recently have been blamed for various health conditions including heart disease, diabetes, and cancer. History shows that our ancestors foraged the land, fished, and hunted wild game, which provided them with an abundant amount of saturated fats, and yet they didn't suffer from these diseases.

As you may have guessed, the fats consumed by our ancestors aren't the same fats we consume today. Again, the change in the fat quality has been impacted by the food we offer the animals: namely, processed grain meal with additives.

Animals are the primary source of our dietary fat. Throughout history, the saturated fat of cattle contained healthy anti-inflammatory compounds, fat-soluble vitamins, and health-boosting conjugated linoleic acid (CLA). These elements were derived from the grass they consumed. Today, the grain-based diet given to cattle on CAFO farms causes their meat to lack these vital components. Instead, the saturated fat of grain-fed cows contains dangerous trans fats, along with antibiotic and hormone residues.

Cholesterol

Cholesterol is a specific type of saturated fat often labeled as unhealthy and dangerous. However, for our body to function optimally, it actually requires cholesterol.

Cholesterol:

- provides structural integrity to our cell membranes
- helps regulate what molecules enter and exit the cell
- is vital for communication between cells and the central nervous system
- surrounds both the central nervous system and brain in a protective case
- is a vital ingredient for the maturation of the brain and nervous system of infants and children
- is a primary ingredient in all the hormones in our bodies

- is a fundamental component of bile, which helps to digest fats
- synthesizes vitamin D in our body
- optimizes immune function

Perhaps the answer to this dilemma is obvious. If we expect to gain the health benefits of wholesome saturated fats, including anti-inflammatory compounds, fat-soluble vitamins, and linoleic acid, we must be aware of where the meat we eat is being raised and what it is being fed. Choosing grass-fed or pasture-raised animals, wild-caught fish, and tropical coconut and palm fats will provide us with cleaner, healthier forms of cholesterol and saturated fats.

UNSATURATED FATS

Unsaturated fats, although considered more beneficial than saturated fats, introduce their own set of problems. This group of fat includes the polyunsaturated omega-3 and omega-6 fats, as well as the monounsaturated omega-9 fats.

Omega-3 Fatty Acids

Omega-3 fatty acids are essential, but the body doesn't produce them; therefore, you must consume them. Fish and seafood are the only direct sources of omega-3 fats. Our bodies can use walnuts, flaxseed, and chia seeds to obtain the precursor for omega-3 fatty acids, but the process of converting it to anti-inflammatory fatty acids takes time, which is not ideal.

Omega-6 Fatty Acids

Omega-6 fatty acids are also considered essential fatty acids because we don't manufacture them, so we must consume them. The primary sources of omega-6 fats are plant oils such as corn, safflower, soybean, cottonseed, sunflower, peanut, grapeseed, and vegetable oils. Since animals on CAFO farms are fed grain-based diets, they have an abundance of omega-6 fatty acids in their meat, which is not helpful.

Omega-9 Fatty Acids

We obtain monounsaturated omega-9 fatty acids from olives, olive oil, avocado, and various nuts and seeds. This is not considered an essential fatty acid, because our body can produce omega-9 fatty acids if our diet doesn't contain adequate amounts.

Omega-3, omega-6, and omega-9 fatty acids must be maintained at a correct balance in our body for optimal health.

FATS AND INFLAMMATION

As we learned earlier, inflammation is a large factor in many chronic health conditions. Balancing omega-6 and omega-3 fats can significantly influence our body's inflammatory response.

Pro-Inflammatory Omega-6 Fatty Acids

The omega-6 fatty acids obtained from eating meat raised on a CAFO farm (especially beef, lamb, or pork) contain a compound called arachidonic acid. This compound is highly inflammatory. Arachidonic acid also comes from refined plant oils including corn, safflower, soybean, cottonseed, sunflower, and peanut. The refining process damages the omega-6 fats, producing arachidonic acid, which increases inflammation. Many of these plants have also been genetically modified, adding another level of concern.

It is also important to know that many imported olive oils have been diluted or "cut" with omega-6 vegetable oils, but this isn't always apparent on the label. This situation is concerning because most individuals consume olive oil because it is healthy. Local olive oil is less likely to be adulterated in this way, but if you can't find local, do your research to make sure the olive oil you purchase is free from rancid, inflammatory vegetable oils.

Anti-Inflammatory Omega-3 Fatty Acids

The typical diet contains an abundance of omega-6 fats but lacks the anti-inflammatory omega-3 fats. Omega-3 fats combat the pro-inflammatory actions of the omega-6 fats. The body converts omega-3 fats into two compounds: eicosapentaenoic acid (EPA) and docosahexaenoic acid (DHA). Both EPA and DHA block arachidonic acid, shutting down the inflammatory pathway.

A few omega-6 fats are considered anti-inflammatory because they assist the omega-3 fat compounds, EPA and DHA, in blocking the inflammatory pathways. They are found in unrefined borage oil, evening primrose oil, and black currant seed oil.

Balancing the pro-inflammatory fats with anti-inflammatory fats is crucial to gut healing. By decreasing the omega-6 to omega-3 ratio to 4:1 from its current status of 25:1 by eating more fish, seafood, chia, and flax seeds and decreasing the pro-inflammatory omega-6 fats, we can control the inflammatory processes that make us so miserable and start healing the gut.

OILS FOR COOKING

There is a lot of confusion regarding which cooking oils are best. Unsaturated fats (omega-3, -6, and -9 fats) are fragile and easily destroyed by heat, air, pressure, and light. Exposure to these elements causes the fats to oxidize, creating free radicals. For this reason, you should avoid using unsaturated fats while cooking. These are best drizzled over cold foods or added to dishes after they have been cooked.

On the other hand, saturated fats are well-organized and resist structural changes from high temperatures. Saturated fats from grass-fed, pastured, or free-range animals and coconut or palm oils provide healthy options. Coconut and palm oils must be unrefined and cold-pressed to retain their healthful properties.

FATS AND *CANDIDA ALBICANS*

Certain fats can inhibit the overgrowth of *Candida albicans* and help maintain a clean gut. Unrefined coconut oil is particularly helpful because of the antifungal compound lauric acid, and it is useful for cooking. The acid in this oil is a very effective antibacterial, antiviral, and antifungal agent. At high concentrations (that is, requiring supplementation), lauric acid effectively kills *Candida albicans*. At lower concentrations, which are found in unrefined coconut oil, lauric acid inhibits the growth of *Candida*, making it a valuable tool for gut healing.

Macadamia oil is another oil that will inhibit *Candida*. As an unsaturated fat and a rich source of palmitoleic acid, an antifungal agent, it makes a particularly healthy salad dressing.

THE BOTTOM LINE FOR GUT HEALING

Fats and oils have the unique ability to heal the gut because they can control inflammation and inhibit common gut infections. It is vital to consume adequate amounts of anti-inflammatory omega-3 fats from seafood or fish oil, as well as indirect sources such as flaxseed oil, chia seeds, and walnut oil. Omega-6 fats from CAFO animals or refined oils can promote inflammation. Refined oils are often rancid and increase the body's free radical burden. Choose omega-6 oils that are cold-pressed and from non-genetically modified plants. Omega-9 fats are another healthy and healing group of oils, supplied by olives and avocados.

Saturated fats from clean sources such as coconut and palm plants and grass-fed animals are an excellent choice for cooking and healing. Unrefined coconut oil supplies therapeutic lauric acid, which inhibits the growth of gut infections. Saturated fats from commercial animals and refined coconut or palm oils are damaging, inducing inflammation and free radical damage.

ELIMINATE COMPLETELY

- Fat from any commercial animal products
- Refined vegetable oils
- Genetically modified oils: vegetable, cottonseed, corn, soybean oil
- Oil or fat alternatives such as shortening, spreadable "butter," and vegan "spreads"

USE SPARINGLY

- Animal fats sourced from grass-fed, pastured, free-range animals

SAFE FATS & OILS

- Cold-pressed extra virgin olive oil (unadulterated brands)
- Unrefined, cold-pressed coconut or palm oil

- Grass-fed butter, if tolerated (contains some casein, but less than any other dairy product)
- Ghee (also known as clarified butter)
- Cold-pressed avocado, macadamia, sesame, walnut, or flaxseed oil

Chapter Summary: Saturated fats are solid, while unsaturated fats are liquid at room temperature. Unsaturated fats include omega-3, -6, and -9 fats. Omega-3 and -6 fats are essential fatty acids because our body can't manufacture them, so we must consume them in our diet. Both influence the body's inflammatory response. Omega-3 fats block the production of inflammatory factors, while most omega-6 fats promote inflammation. Therefore, a healing diet must focus on anti-inflammatory omega-3 fats from seafood and fish oil.

Saturated fats such as coconut and palm oil are best for cooking at high temperatures, while unsaturated, plant-based oils should not be exposed to heat. Coconut oil inhibits the growth of bacteria, viruses, and *Candida albicans* and is therapeutic for the gut.

CHAPTER 20:
FERMENTED FOODS, VINEGAR & ALCOHOL

T HIS CHAPTER EXPLORES THE CONTROVERSIAL topics of fermentation and vinegar in the context of gut healing. There are very logical proofs on both sides of these debates, but after we dissect and eliminate the obvious dilemmas, personal application of the debatable particulars will be different for each person, based on what their body tells them.

DEBATES ON FERMENTATION

Almost everyone agrees that fermented foods are healthy, but not everyone can agree on whether fermented foods are acceptable in the presence of gut infections. Old-school *Candida* diets forbid the consumption of all fermented foods, including alcohol, sauerkraut, kimchi, kefir, pickles, and vinegar. Many continue to believe fermented food introduces species of bacteria and yeast and exacerbates gut infections, weakens the immune system, and prevents gut healing. Nonetheless, fermented foods impart beneficial probiotics that can help reestablish a healthy balance of gut bacteria. There is validity to both arguments. Hopefully, I will untangle the confusion and present a position that will promote gut health and healing for all based on your personal circumstances.

FERMENTING FOR HEALTH

Fermentation occurs when bacteria and yeast metabolize sugars into acids, gases, and alcohol. Historically, fermented foods such as sauerkraut, pickles, kimchi, and yogurt were an important component of a healthy diet because it was one of few methods available for food preservation. As bacteria and yeast ferment the carbohydrate molecules in vegetables, fruit, or milk, lactic acid is formed. This healthful acid not only preserves food from dangerous bacteria but also aids in digestion. As the natural enzymes and acids pre-digest nutrients, vitamins and minerals become more available for absorption. Other compounds produced through fermentation can scavenge damaging free radicals and act as antioxidants.

The lactic acid bacteria present in fermented foods possess several health-promoting characteristics. Not only do they support digestion and increase nutrient availability, but they produce enzymes that help destroy and eliminate toxins. Lactic acid bacteria protect cells from damage and encourage cell growth and reproduction.[114] They exhibit antimicrobial activities that inhibit infectious organisms such as *Listeria, S. aureus, E. coli* and *Salmonella*.[115] This activity is especially strong in fermented vegetables such as kimchi, a spicy Korean fermented cabbage dish.

Studies confirm lactic acid bacteria are helpful in improving common gastrointestinal disorders such as inflammatory bowel disease, ulcerative colitis, and acute diarrhea. *Lactobacillus*, one of the bacterial strains isolated from kefir and kimchi, protects against allergic reactions and increases the body's tolerance to potential allergens.

With so many health-promoting benefits, it seems unreasonable to recommend that everyone eliminate fermented foods simply because they contain yeast and bacteria. Still, despite the obvious benefits, everyone's body responds differently to the microbes introduced through fermentation. Therefore, if your body doesn't seem to heal with fermented foods, I suggest you eliminate them and reevaluate your progress. If you do choose to include fermented foods, I still recommend avoiding fermented dairy such as kefir and yogurt: casein remains problematic for gut health. Coconut or water kefir is a better option for gut healing.

VINEGAR

Traditionally, vinegar has been eliminated during gut healing and especially when *Candida* infections exist. But recently, the promotion of raw apple cider vinegar for health has raised the question of whether vinegar might be acceptable as part of a healing diet. Current research supports the use of raw apple cider vinegar, which may help kill specific gut infections, but all other forms of vinegar are not helpful for gut health.

The controversy of vinegar focuses on its influence over the body's pH. Raw apple cider vinegar is uniquely alkaline-forming in the body, but all other kinds of vinegar increase the body's acidity. *Candida* and other harmful organisms thrive in an acidic environment. To inhibit the growth of these organisms, you must establish an alkaline environment. Eliminating acid-forming vinegar is necessary for maintaining an alkaline pH. Since many condiments such as mustard, ketchup, mayonnaise, and dressings include white vinegar, you must eliminate them from a gut-healing diet unless you can find vinegar-free varieties.

Even though raw apple cider vinegar is alkalinizing and may help eradicate infections, some individuals still experience negative symptoms associated with *Candida* when consuming raw apple cider vinegar.[116] If you are among this group, I suggest you avoid all vinegar and replace it with lemon juice. Observing your own body's response to foods is important and should always be the final determinant in whether you choose to consume a generally "acceptable" item or avoid it.

ALCOHOL

Alcoholic beverages contain unhealthy yeast that exacerbates *Candida* infections, and the alcoholic content itself disrupts the gut microbiota. When alcohol comes into contact with the cells of the small intestine, it disrupts the communication between the gut bacteria and the immune system. It first damages the intestinal cells and then begins to destroy the immune cells in the gut. Once it succeeds at weakening the immune system, the mucosal gut barrier becomes permeable, establishing leaky gut.[117] As we learned earlier, a leaky gut allows infectious organisms to pass into the bloodstream, activating the immune system, establishing inflammation, and further destroying the gut.

Even small amounts of alcohol burden the liver as it works to detox toxins from the body. Infections in the gut leak biotoxins into the bloodstream, and the liver is responsible for cleaning these up. When alcohol induces an inflammatory response in the gut, it weakens the liver's ability to detox. Clearly, alcohol is not your friend as you attempt to heal your gut. It is counterproductive to healing, as it strains the gut, immune system, and liver.

As an important side note, many healthy fermented drinks such as kombucha and kvass contain small amounts of alcohol (averaging 0.5 percent). In some cases, the health-promoting acids and microbes negate the potential effects of the alcohol. However, as with fermented foods and vinegar, if you feel kombucha is not helping you heal, then eliminate it. In advanced cases of dysbiosis and leaky gut, even the smallest amount of alcohol can hinder healing.

THE BOTTOM LINE FOR GUT HEALING

Fermented foods certainly come with an abundance of health-promoting advantages. They supply the gut with healthy acids that help alkalinize the body, digestive enzymes, antioxidants, beneficial bacteria, and immune-boosting nutrients. Yet there will still be some individuals with very advanced cases of leaky gut who will not find fermented foods to be helpful and who would do well to avoid them. If you do experience benefits, you should still limit your choices of fermented foods to fermented vegetables only. Fermented fruit contains more yeast than vegetables, which impart more health-boosting lactic acid bacteria.

Vinegar influences the body's acidity. Raw apple cider vinegar possesses unique acids that act to alkalinize the body, but all other forms of vinegar are highly acidic and lack live enzymes and acids. You should avoid these, as harmful yeast and bacteria thrive in an acidic body.

Alcohol disrupts the gut microbiota and burdens the liver's ability to detox the body. It is best if you avoid all alcohol while you heal your gut.

ELIMINATE COMPLETELY

- All alcoholic beverages
- Cooking wines and vinegar
- All vinegar, except raw apple cider vinegar
- Condiments containing vinegar
- Fermented fruit

USE SPARINGLY

- Raw apple cider vinegar
- Kombucha (fermented tea) or kvass, if tolerated

SAFE FERMENTED FOODS & VINEGAR REPLACEMENTS

- Lemon or lime juice replaces vinegar in any recipe
- Coconut aminos replace soy sauce
- Fermented vegetables such as sauerkraut, kimchi, pickles (look for preservative-free varieties or homemade)
- Coconut or water kefir

Chapter Summary: Fermented foods impart many healthy benefits and can be part of a gut-healing diet; however, it is imperative to eliminate alcohol and vinegar (except raw apple cider vinegar).

PART 3:

THE DIET & NUTRACEUTICAL PLAN
HOW DOES THIS WORK?

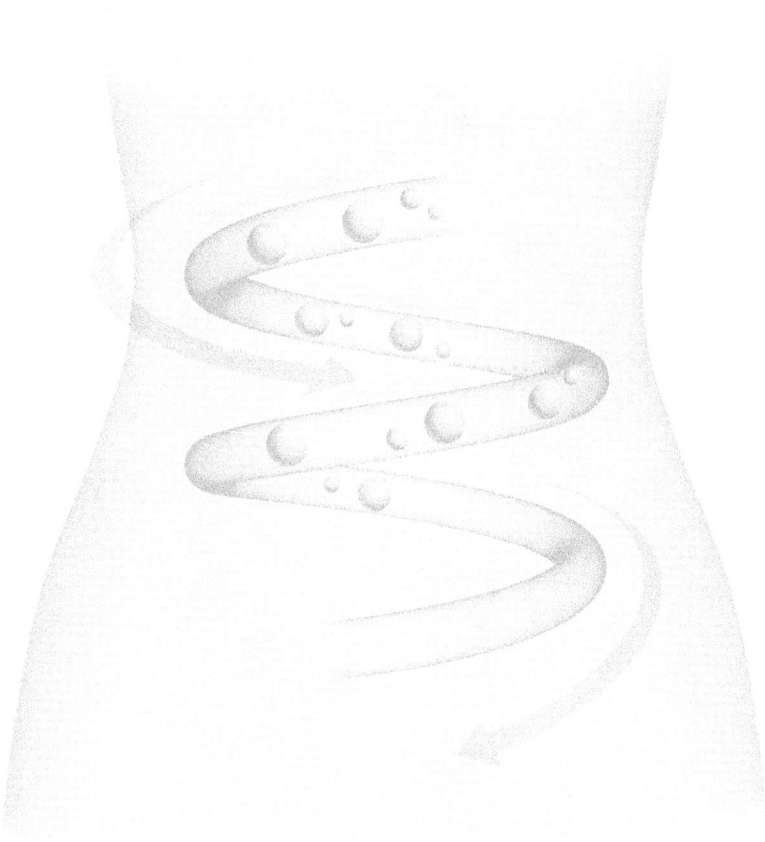

THE DIET & NUTRACEUTICAL PLAN

Now that you understand why it is so important to begin your journey toward lifelong health with the gut, and how food heals the gut, it is time to look at how this works in practice. In this section, I provide you with a four-week meal plan that can be used for all stages of your gut-healing journey.

You may have to follow this plan for up to a year, depending on your state of health and your age. Each day includes an ideal amount of protein, carbohydrates, and fat. All meals include a grain-free option to accommodate those who choose to eliminate grains temporarily. This meal plan does not eliminate FODMAPS, so if you find that you need to eliminate these, feel free to substitute vegetables as required.

How to Use the Menu Plan

This meal plan is designed to be convenient and cost-effective to serve the most readers. I don't attempt to include gourmet meals or ingredients that would be difficult to find. Additionally, I utilize leftovers and attempt to stretch ingredients over several meals.

Don't feel constrained by the menu plan. For example, you will notice that I use eggs for breakfast many days. They are easy and inexpensive while providing an excellent source of healthy fat and protein. However, I would encourage you to use protein shakes at least three days a week in place of eggs, or to experiment with other breakfast recipes found in this book but not used in the menu plan.

The meals are very versatile and almost any vegetable, meat, or fruit can be substituted for a similar item in the same food group. Feel free to replace recipes with your own favorites if they agree with the gut-healing principles you've learned in this book. Be creative and enjoy your customizable menu plan.

When cooking meats, you will find that I will attempt to utilize the meat or broth in several ways. For example, if you roast a whole chicken in the oven, you can pull off the meat and use it for a few meals while reusing the carcass to make bone broth. If you review the meals for the week, you will discover how I stretch both the meat and the broth.

The Recipes

Recipes from this book are indicated with an asterisk (*) in the meal plans. You will find the recipes in Part 4. You will also notice additional recipes in each section that may not appear in the menu plan. These recipes are for those who may not be governed by convenience or cost, or who desire variety. Although they are not in the menu plan, they are nourishing and gut-healing. I also provide ideas and recipes for snacks, beverages, and special desserts in Part 4.

Most of the recipes are designed to feed a family of four, so you may have to adjust the quantity according to your needs. If you have a very busy schedule, I recommend making extra quantities and freezing as many portions as you can.

I make all the recipes found in this book regularly in my home, so here I offer you a glimpse into my own eating style, and I can promise they will be tasty, yet convenient. Although I don't follow a menu plan, I can attest that it saves time when you get into the habit of making and following one. In my perfect world, I would have a well-stocked freezer and a four-week menu plan. Instead, I offer you one.

If you are like me, pictures inspire you to cook. Browsing through colorful, pictorial recipe books is a pastime of mine. If you want to see photos of any of the recipes in this book, go to my website at **www.purelifehw.com/ recipes** to find those inspiring photos.

Nutraceutical Plan

This menu plan is also accompanied by a nutraceutical schedule that will help you organize the best supportive supplements and take them at the most ideal times.

Resources

Finally, you will find helpful resources for how to purchase food and supplements online. I find it much less expensive to purchase quality, nonperishable items through an online retailer rather than a health food store. Many of these same retailers can provide the supplements you need. I don't make specific supplement recommendations because manufacturers are constantly changing their formulas and doing so would require constant updates. I only use a few selected professional-grade supplement companies for my clients, making it impossible to review all the options available.

WEEK 1			
	BREAKFAST	**LUNCH**	**DINNER**
MONDAY	Morning Shake* or 2-3 sautéed eggs + ½ avocado + sautéed kale topped with salsa	Chicken Curry Salad* on celery sticks	Mexican Taco Salad*
TUESDAY	Morning Shake* or 2-3 sautéed eggs + Sauerkraut* + 1 citrus fruit	leftover Chicken Curry Salad* on lettuce	Grilled Salmon* + sautéed zucchini + Cauliflower Rice* (or Baked Brown Rice*)
WEDNESDAY	Morning Shake* or Coconut Paleo Pancakes* + nut butter	Marinated Vegetable Salad* in a jar	Chicken Fennel Stir Fry* over Zucchini Noodles* (or shirataki noodles or quinoa)
THURSDAY	Morning Shake* or 2-3 scrambled eggs + green onions and fresh parsley + Sauerkraut*	leftover Chicken Fennel Stir Fry* over lettuce + avocado + extra virgin olive oil	Robust Chili*
FRIDAY	Morning Shake* or 2-3 hardboiled eggs + 2 sugar-free bacon + sautéed kale.	leftover Robust Chili*	Roasted chicken + stir fry veggies + sesame seeds (quinoa, opt.)
SATURDAY	Brunch: Veggie Frittata* + citrus fruit	Grilled Chicken Fennel Salad*	
SUNDAY	leftover Veggie Frittata*	Salmon Patties* + veggies + hummus	Quick One Pot Roast*

* Recipe found in Part 4

	BREAKFAST	LUNCH	DINNER
WEEK 2			
MONDAY	Morning Shake* or Easy Egg Muffins*	leftover Quick One Pot Roast* over lettuce	Almond Crusted White Fish* + Basic Coleslaw* + baked sweet potato (topped with coconut butter, cinnamon, flaxseed)
TUESDAY	Morning Shake* or 2-3 sautéed eggs + Sauerkraut* + sautéed onion/ pepper	leftover sweet potato (topped with coconut butter, cinnamon, flaxseed) + Basic Coleslaw*	One Pot Chicken Curry* over spaghetti squash "noodles" (or Baked Brown Rice*)
WEDNESDAY	Morning Shake* or Coconut Paleo Pancakes* + nut butter	Marinated Vegetable Salad* in a jar	Chicken Fennel Stir Fry* over zucchini noodles (or shirataki or quinoa)
THURSDAY	Morning Shake* or Easy Egg Muffins*	leftover Chicken Fennel Stir Fry* over lettuce	Chicken Italiano Salad*
FRIDAY	Morning Shake* or 2-3 scrambled eggs + parsley, green onions + Sauerkraut*	Marinated Vegetable Salad* in a jar (add leftover chicken and cooked quinoa)	Detox Green Soup*
SATURDAY	Brunch: Paleo Pumpkin Pancakes* + Homemade Breakfast Sausage* + Sauerkraut*	Salmon Taco Bowls*	
SUNDAY	Morning Glory Muffins* + sugar-free bacon	leftover Detox Green Soup*	Paleo "Hobo" Dinner*

* Recipe found in Part 4

WEEK 3			
	BREAKFAST	**LUNCH**	**DINNER**
MONDAY	Morning Shake* or 2-3 sautéed eggs + ½ avocado + sautéed kale Top with salsa.	Salmon Patties* + Sauerkraut* + tomato slices	One Pot Chicken Curry* over spaghetti squash "noodles" (or Baked Brown Rice*)
TUESDAY	Morning Shake* or Apple Cinnamon Muffins* + sugar-free bacon	Marinated Vegetable Salad* in a jar (add leftover chicken)	Grass-fed hamburgers + Sweet Curried Broccoli Salad* + Vegetable "Fries"*
WEDNESDAY	Morning Shake* or Coconut Paleo Pancakes* + nut butter	leftover Sweet Curried Broccoli Salad* + pumpkin seeds	Almond Crusted White Fish* + Creamy Avocado Dressing* + Tropical Cabbage Salad*
THURSDAY	Morning Shake* or Morning Glory Muffins*	Hard-boiled eggs + veggie slices + hummus	Chicken Burrito Bowls*
FRIDAY	Morning Shake* or 2-3 hard-boiled eggs + Sauerkraut*	Sautéed cabbage, black beans, tomatoes, salsa, cilantro (from leftover taco salad)	Asian Meatballs* + Zucchini "noodles"*
SATURDAY	Brunch: Veggie Omelets* + Homemade Breakfast Sausage*	Chicken Italiano Salad* + gut-healing dessert of choice	
SUNDAY	Paleo Pumpkin Pancakes* + nut butter + berries	Refreshing Power Greens Salad* + leftover Asian Meatballs*	Spicy Chicken Soup*

* Recipe found in Part 4

WEEK 4

	BREAKFAST	LUNCH	DINNER
MONDAY	Morning Shake* or 2-3 scrambled eggs + parsley, green onions + Sauerkraut*	leftover Spicy Chicken Soup*	Sesame Orange Salmon* over sautéed cabbage + citrus fruit slices
TUESDAY	Morning Shake* or Apple Cinnamon Muffins* + sugar-free bacon	Chicken Curry Salad* on celery sticks	Quick One Pot Roast* + Refreshing Power Greens Salad*
WEDNESDAY	Morning Shake* or Zucchini Pancakes* + low sugar fruit	Chicken Curry Salad* on lettuce + carrots	Detox Green Soup*
THURSDAY	Morning Shake* Or 2-3 sautéed eggs + ½ avocado + sautéed kale topped with salsa	Leftover Detox Green Soup*	Roasted Chicken* + stir fried veggies + quinoa (optional)
FRIDAY	Morning Shake* or Morning Glory Muffins*	Leftover Roasted Chicken* + stir fried veggies over lettuce	Mexican Taco Salad*
SATURDAY	Brunch: Veggie Omelets* + Homemade Breakfast Sausage*	Paleo Hobo Dinner*	
SUNDAY	Paleo Pumpkin Pancakes* + nut butter + berries	Cruciferous Cocktail Salad*	Almond Crusted White Fish* + green beans + acorn squash topped with coconut butter, cinnamon, and flaxseed

* Recipe found in Part 4

SUGGESTED NUTRACEUTICAL SCHEDULE

	BREAKFAST		LUNCH		DINNER		BEDTIME
	30-min. before	During	30-min. before	During	30-min. before	During	
Antimicrobial	X		X		X		
Biofilm "busters"	X		X		X		
Digestive Enzymes, Betaine HCl		X		X		X	
Probiotics							X
L-Glutamine		X					
Omega-3 fatty acids		X					
Zinc		X					
Vitamin D		X					
Gut-soothing herbs (DGL, aloe vera, marshmallow, quercetin, etc.)	X — As needed		X — As needed		X — As needed		

PART 4:

THE RESOURCES

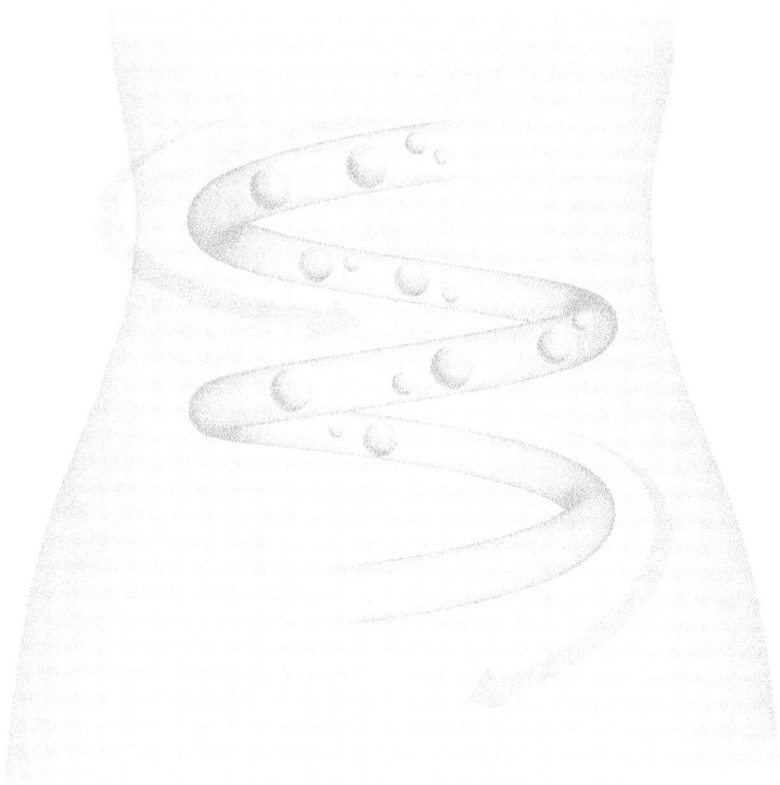

CORE RECIPES

CREAMY AVOCADO DRESSING

Makes 2 cups

- » 1 avocado, pitted
- » ½ cup homemade mayonnaise (see recipe on page 229)
- » ½ cup canned unsweetened coconut milk
- » 1 tablespoon lemon juice, or raw apple cider vinegar
- » 2 cloves garlic
- » 1 sprig green onion
- » 2 tablespoons fresh cilantro
- » 2 tablespoons fresh parsley
- » 1 tablespoon fresh dill, or 1 teaspoon dried dill
- » ½ teaspoon salt
- » ½ teaspoon pepper

Instructions

1. Mix all ingredients in a blender.
2. Blend well and store extra in the refrigerator for 5 to 7 days.

BASIC ALMOND MILK

Makes 6 cups

- » 2 cups raw almonds
- » 12 cups filtered water, divided
- » 1 tablespoon pure vanilla extract
- » pinch sea salt
- » ½ teaspoon powdered stevia, or 7 to 10 drops of liquid stevia (optional)

Instructions

1. Soak almonds in at least 4 cups of water for 12 hours.
2. Drain water and rinse almonds well.
3. Place almonds in a blender with 8 cups of filtered water.
4. Blend on high for 2 to 3 minutes.
5. Line a strainer with cheesecloth and place the strainer over a large glass measuring bowl.
6. Slowly pour the blended almond mixture into the cheesecloth, stirring with a spoon to help separate the liquid from the almond meal.
7. When the last bit of liquid is poured into the cheesecloth, squeeze the cheesecloth to remove any excess liquid (reserve the almond meal for future recipes).
8. Pour the strained liquid back into the blender.
9. Add the vanilla, sea salt, and stevia (optional) and blend for 30 seconds.
10. Pour into a glass container and refrigerate for up to 7 days.

CLARIFIED BUTTER (CASEIN-FREE BUTTER)

Makes 1 pound

» 1 pound of grass-fed butter (I recommend Kerrygold brand)

Instructions

1. Melt the butter in a saucepan on low heat.

2. Skim the milk solids (casein) that rise to the top in a foamy mixture.

3. Strain the remaining butter through cheesecloth, into a glass container. Store in the refrigerator for up to 1 year.

Note: If you allow the butter to cook longer, the milk solids will turn brown and fall to the bottom. You can then strain the butter through cheesecloth. This is called ghee. It will store at room temperature for up to 3 months.

GUT-HEALING BONE BROTH

Makes ~ 1 gallon

- » 1 chicken or turkey carcass (from a roasted chicken with the meat pulled off), or 2 to 3 raw beef shank or large knuckle bones
- » 1 to 2 gallons filtered water
- » 2 tablespoons raw apple cider vinegar
- » 1 tablespoon sea salt

Optional add-ins for higher mineral content:

- » 5 to 6 cloves garlic, coarsely minced
- » 1 onion, chopped roughly
- » 2 to 3 carrots, chopped roughly
- » 2 to 3 celery stalks, chopped roughly
- » 2 to 3 handfuls of fresh herbs (parsley, dill, cilantro, basil, oregano, etc.)
- » 1 teaspoon dried turmeric

Instructions

1. Place bones in a large slow cooker.
2. Cover with filtered water.
3. Add salt, vinegar, and any additional vegetables or spices.
4. Fill the remainder of the slow cooker with filtered water.
5. Cook on high for 12 to 24 hours.
6. Store broth in the refrigerator for no more than 2 to 3 days. Freeze remaining broth.

Note: If you have an Instant Pot or pressure cooker, you can cook on high pressure for 2 hours.

GUACAMOLE

Makes 1 cup

- » 1 soft avocado
- » ¼ teaspoon sea salt
- » ½ teaspoon lemon juice
- » ⅛ teaspoon black pepper
- » ¼ teaspoon onion powder
- » ¼ teaspoon garlic powder
- » ¼ teaspoon curry powder or turmeric and cumin

Instructions

1. Mash avocado with a fork.
2. Add all remaining ingredients and mix well.
3. Store in the refrigerator for 2 to 3 days in an airtight container.

Note: Different seasonings can be added to the guacamole, to add variety.

GREEK SALAD DRESSING

Makes 1 cup

- » Juice of 2 lemons or ¼ cup preservative-free lemon juice
- » ½ extra virgin olive oil
- » 2 cloves garlic
- » 1 ½ tablespoon dried oregano or 4 tablespoons fresh oregano
- » 1 tablespoon dried basil or 3 tablespoons fresh basil
- » 1 teaspoon sea salt
- » ½ teaspoon black pepper

Instructions

1. Mix all in a blender until well combined.
2. Store in the refrigerator for up to 1 week.

Note: This can be used as a chicken or beef marinade.

GUT HEALING MAYO

Makes 1 cup

- » 2 egg yolks
- » 1 tablespoon lemon juice
- » ½ teaspoon sea salt
- » ½ teaspoon onion powder
- » ½ teaspoon garlic powder
- » ½ teaspoon ground mustard seed
- » ¼ teaspoon black pepper
- » 1 cup avocado oil or a similar light-tasting oil

Instructions

1. Using a hand mixer or blender, whisk (or blend on low) egg yolks, lemon juice, and spices until almost fluffy.

2. Slowly add oil a few drops at a time, whisking constantly. Slowly drizzle the oil into the mixture during the last ½ cup.

3. Store mayonnaise in the refrigerator for up to 2 weeks.

Note: You may make a spicier version by adding cayenne pepper, chili powder, cumin, turmeric or other spices to suite your taste. Replacing some oil with melted bacon fat provides another tasty option.

SAUERKRAUT

Makes 1 gallon

- » 3 heads cabbage, shredded (retain 2 to 3 whole cabbage leaves)
- » 3 tablespoons sea salt
- » 3 to 4 slices onion
- » 3-4 carrots, shredded (optional)
- » 1 tablespoon caraway seeds (optional)

Instructions

1. Place all ingredients in a large bowl and sprinkle salt on top.
2. Using clean hands, squeeze and massage the mixture for 3 to 5 minutes, or until the mixture has produced a large amount of liquid.
3. Pack the mixture into a gallon size glass jar, pressing down tightly to reduce air space and bring the liquid to the top.
4. If the liquid does not cover the top, add some filtered water.
5. Arrange the onion slices on top.
6. Cover the cabbage mixture with whole cabbage leaves (ripping slightly so they lie flat).
7. Place a ceramic or glass bowl on top of the cabbage leaves and fill with water, to hold down the mixture.
8. Cover with a loose lid, if possible.
9. Ferment 3 to 7 days on the countertop or in your pantry.
10. Store in the refrigerator for up to 1 month. The flavor will intensify with time.

Note: Make sure the sauerkraut is covered in liquid. Any exposed sauerkraut may develop mold. If this happens, throw away the top layer of sauerkraut. Also, *do not* use any metal utensils when working with fermented foods!

BREAKFAST RECIPES

Morning Shake

Makes 1 serving

- » 1 handful dark leafy greens
- » ½ cup low-sugar frozen fruit
- » 1 scoop protein powder
- » ½ cup or 1 small handful of a dietary fat (full fat coconut milk, nuts, avocado)
- » Liquid, as needed (water, coconut water, nut milk)
- » Optional add-ins (fish oil, chia seeds, herbs, powdered nutraceuticals)

Instructions

1. Place all ingredients into a high-powered blender, in the order presented.
2. Blend on high until smooth.

APPLE CINNAMON MUFFINS

Makes 12 muffins

- » 3 large green apples, diced small
- » 3 tablespoons water
- » 9 eggs
- » 3 tablespoons unsweetened coconut milk
- » 1 ½ tablespoons unrefined coconut oil, melted
- » 1 teaspoon cinnamon
- » 1 teaspoon powdered stevia (I recommend Stevita Supreme or SweetLeaf brand)
- » 2 tablespoons coconut flour
- » ½ teaspoon baking soda
- » ¼ teaspoon sea salt

Instructions

1. Preheat oven to 350 degrees.
2. Oil a muffin pan with coconut oil or prepare with liners.
3. Heat a large skillet on medium-high heat.
4. Add apples and water, and cover.
5. Cook apples until softened. Set aside.
6. In a medium-sized bowl, whisk eggs.
7. Add remaining ingredients and mix well.
8. Add apples and combine.
9. Divide batter between muffin cups.
10. Bake for 40 minutes or until muffins are firm.
11. Store extra in the refrigerator for up to 1 week or freeze.

BERRY COBBLER

Makes 6 servings

- » 4 cups fresh blackberries, raspberries, blueberries, or strawberries, rinsed
- » ½ cup coconut flour
- » ½ cup almond flour or almond meal
- » ¾ teaspoon baking soda
- » ¼ teaspoon salt
- » 1 teaspoon cinnamon
- » 1 teaspoon ginger
- » ¼ teaspoon nutmeg
- » 3 eggs
- » 1 cup coconut milk
- » 1 teaspoon pure vanilla extract
- » 1 teaspoon lemon juice
- » 1 teaspoon powdered stevia (I recommend Stevita Supreme or SweetLeaf brand)

Instructions

1. Preheat oven to 325 degrees.
2. Grease an 8x8 glass baking dish with coconut oil.
3. Arrange the berries in the baking dish.
4. Combine all the remaining ingredients and mix well until a smooth batter forms.
5. Pour the batter over the berries and smooth out with a spatula.
6. Bake for 35-45 minutes or until the batter is firm to touch.
7. Serve warm.
8. Store extra in the refrigerator for up to 1 week in an airtight container.

COCONUT PALEO PANCAKES

Makes 8 small pancakes

- » 4 tablespoons unrefined coconut oil
- » ½ cup coconut flour
- » ½ teaspoon baking soda
- » 1 teaspoon cinnamon
- » 4 tablespoons natural almond butter
- » 4 eggs
- » 1 teaspoon powdered stevia (I recommend Stevita Supreme or SweetLeaf brand)
- » ½ cup almond or coconut milk
- » ¼ cup ground flaxseed (optional)
- » 2 cups frozen berries
- » 1 tablespoon water

Instructions

1. Heat 2 tablespoons of coconut oil in a large skillet on medium heat.
2. Mix all ingredients until well blended.
3. Pour batter onto hot skillet, cooking until bubbles appear on the top of the pancakes.
4. Flip pancakes and cook on the other side.
5. Add more coconut oil to the skillet, as needed, for remaining pancakes.
6. In a small saucepan, heat berries and water.
7. Lightly mash the berries a few times, leaving some whole.
8. Serve pancakes with berries poured on top.

DETOX EGGS BENEDICT

Makes 2 servings

- » 2-3 tablespoons unrefined coconut oil
- » 1 cup purple or green cabbage, shredded
- » ½ cup zucchini, chopped
- » 1 tablespoon fresh parsley, chopped
- » 1 tablespoon fresh cilantro, chopped
- » sea salt, to taste
- » ½ teaspoon turmeric
- » ¼ teaspoon onion powder
- » 3 eggs
- » 1-2 tablespoons coconut milk
- » salt, to taste
- » black pepper, to taste
- » 1 teaspoon garlic, minced

Instructions

1. Heat coconut oil in a large skillet on medium heat.
2. Sauté cabbage and zucchini, leaving slightly crisp.
3. Add parsley, cilantro, salt, turmeric and onion powder to the skillet and stir.
4. In a small bowl, whisk eggs, coconut milk, pepper, salt and garlic.
5. Pour egg mixture over the vegetables.
6. Place a lid on the skillet and let eggs harden, stirring occasionally.

EASY EGG MUFFINS

Makes 12 muffins

- » 1 tablespoon unrefined coconut oil
- » 12 eggs
- » ½ pound sausage, bacon, or leftover meat, cooked and diced
- » 2 cups veggies, diced (any combination)
- » ¼ teaspoon sea salt
- » ⅛ teaspoon black pepper
- » 3 tablespoons water

Instructions

1. Preheat oven to 350 degrees.
2. Oil each muffin cup with coconut oil or line with paper.
3. Whisk eggs in a medium bowl.
4. Add remaining ingredients and mix well.
5. Divide batter between muffin cups.
6. Bake for 20 minutes or until middle is firm.
7. Serve warm.

Note: These muffins freeze and reheat very well for a quick breakfast or snack. Additional seasonings can be added for variety and flavor.

HOMEMADE BREAKFAST SAUSAGE

Makes 6 patties

- » 1 pound ground pork, turkey, chicken, or beef
- » 1 teaspoon dried sage
- » ½ teaspoon onion powder
- » ½ teaspoon garlic powder
- » ½ teaspoon dried thyme
- » 1 teaspoon fennel seeds
- » 1 teaspoon sea salt
- » ¼ teaspoon black pepper

Instructions

1. Heat a large skillet over medium heat.
2. Combine all ingredients and mix well.
3. Form patties with clean hands.
4. Cook patties approximately 8 minutes on each side.

Note: If you use ground chicken or turkey, you may have to add some coconut oil to your skillet. Make several batches and freeze cooked or uncooked patties for future meals.

MORNING GLORY MUFFINS (GRAIN-FREE)

Makes 2 dozen

- » 1 cup mashed squash, sweet potato, or pumpkin
- » 4 eggs, beaten
- » 1 teaspoon pure vanilla extract
- » 1 teaspoon pure orange extract (optional)
- » 1 cup zucchini, grated and squeezed to remove extra liquid
- » 1 cup green apples, grated
- » 1 cup carrots, grated
- » 1 ½ cups fine-ground almond flour
- » ½ cup coconut flour
- » ½ cup flaxmeal
- » 1 cup unsweetened shredded coconut
- » 2/3 cup walnuts, chopped (or other nuts)
- » 1 tablespoon powdered stevia (I recommend Stevita Supreme or SweetLeaf brand)
- » 1 teaspoon ginger
- » 2 teaspoons cinnamon
- » 1 teaspoon baking powder
- » ½ teaspoon baking soda
- » ½ teaspoon sea salt

Instructions

1. Preheat oven to 350 degrees.
2. Line or oil a muffin tin.

3. In a large bowl, combine squash, eggs, extracts, zucchini, apples, and carrots.

4. In a medium bowl, combine remaining (dry) ingredients.

5. Combine wet and dry ingredients and mix well.

6. Divide batter between muffin pans.

7. Bake for 30-35 minutes or until firm.

8. Cool on a wire rack before removing muffins from pan.

9. Freeze extra muffins.

Note: The batter will be very thick and the texture of these "muffins" is dense. You may add additional eggs if you desire a lighter muffin.

PALEO PUMPKIN PANCAKES

Makes 12-15 pancakes

- » 8 eggs
- » 1 cup canned pure pumpkin puree
- » 2 teaspoons powdered stevia (I recommend Stevita Supreme or SweetLeaf brand)
- » 2 teaspoons pure vanilla extract
- » 2 teaspoons cinnamon
- » 1 teaspoon nutmeg
- » 1 teaspoon ginger
- » 1 ½ teaspoon baking soda
- » ½ teaspoon sea salt
- » 4 tablespoons coconut flour
- » 4-5 tablespoons unrefined coconut oil

Instructions

1. Whisk eggs in a medium bowl.
2. Add remaining ingredients and mix well.
3. Heat a large skillet on medium heat.
4. Add 2 tablespoons of coconut oil and spoon batter into skillet.
5. Flip each pancake when bubbles appear on the surface.
6. Add more coconut oil, as needed.

VEGGIE OMELETS

Makes 1

- » 2 eggs
- » 1 tablespoon of coconut fat from the top of a can of coconut milk
- » pinch of sea salt
- » pinch of black pepper
- » 1 tablespoon unrefined coconut oil
- » 1 cup chopped vegetables (peppers, onions, garlic, spinach, swiss chard, arugula, zucchini, tomatoes, fresh spices)
- » 2 tablespoons sugar-free salsa
- » 1 tablespoon homemade mayonnaise (recipe on page 229) or avocado ranch dressing (recipe on page 223)

Instructions

1. Heat an 8-inch skillet over medium to low heat.
2. Whisk egg, coconut fat, sea salt and pepper.
3. Add coconut oil to skillet.
4. Pour egg mixture into skillet and start swirling eggs with a heat-resistant spatula.
5. After eggs begin to solidify, place lid on omelet, reduce heat to low, and let sit for 2 to 3 minutes or until eggs are set.
6. Spread chopped vegetables over half the omelet.
7. Place salsa, mayo or dressing on top of vegetables and use the spatula to fold the omelet.
8. Slide onto a plate.

VEGETABLE FRITTATA

Makes 6 servings

- » 2 tablespoons unrefined coconut oil
- » 1 onion
- » 3 cloves garlic, minced
- » 3 cups vegetables of your choice
- » 12 eggs
- » 2 tablespoons coconut fat (skimmed from the top of canned coconut milk) or ¼ cup water
- » 1 teaspoon oregano
- » 1 teaspoon basil
- » 1 teaspoon sea salt
- » ½ teaspoon black pepper

Instructions

1. Using a large cast-iron (or oven-safe) skillet, heat the coconut oil on medium heat.
2. Add onion and sauté for 2 minutes.
3. Add remaining vegetables and spices and sauté for 2-3 minutes, leaving vegetables slightly crisp.
4. In a medium bowl, whisk eggs and coconut fat or water.
5. Pour eggs over the vegetables in the skillet.
6. Stir a few times to let the eggs settle on the bottom of the skillet.
7. Turn the heat to medium low and turn the oven on low broil.
8. Place a lid on the skillet and wait for 5 minutes.

9. Gently lift the lid to see if the eggs are set around the edges. Only the middle should still have soft eggs. If not, replace the lid and continue cooking until sides are set.

10. Place the cast-iron skillet under the broiler and broil until the eggs are completely set on top.

11. Serve immediately.

Note: Leftovers can be frozen as individual slices and reheated later.

ZUCCHINI PANCAKES

Makes 8 pancakes

- » 2 tablespoons unrefined coconut oil
- » 3 eggs
- » 2 cups shredded zucchini
- » 1 tablespoon coconut flour
- » ¼ teaspoon sea salt
- » ¼ teaspoon black pepper

Instructions

1. Heat coconut oil in a large skillet on medium-low heat.
2. Place zucchini in a strainer and squeeze out excess water (or squeeze with a paper towel).
3. Whisk eggs in a medium bowl.
4. Add zucchini and remaining ingredients and mix well.
5. Spoon batter onto the hot skillet to make pancakes.
6. Cook each side for 4 minutes, until they are firm to touch.

CHICKEN & TURKEY RECIPES

Blueberry Chicken Salad

Makes 4 servings

- » 3 boneless, skinless chicken breasts
- » 2 teaspoons creole seasoning
- » 2 tablespoons unrefined coconut oil
- » 8 cups romaine lettuce, roughly chopped
- » 1 cup fresh berries
- » 1 handful fresh parsley, chopped
- » 1 (15.5oz) can unsweetened coconut milk
- » ¼ cup raw apple cider vinegar or lemon juice
- » 1 teaspoon powdered stevia (I recommend Stevita Supreme or SweetLeaf brand)
- » 1 handful fresh cilantro
- » 1 teaspoon dried basil

Instructions

1. Heat a large skill on medium heat.
2. Coat chicken breasts in coconut oil and creole.
3. Cook chicken in heated skillet until juices run clear.
4. Arrange lettuce, berries and fresh parsley on plates.
5. Combine remaining ingredients in a blender and mix well.
6. Place chicken on top of salads and pour dressing over all.

CHICKEN BURRITO BOWLS (SLOW COOKER)

Makes 4 servings

- » 2 pounds boneless, skinless chicken (any combination of breasts, thighs or leg quarters)
- » 1 onion, diced
- » 4 cloves garlic, minced
- » 1 (8oz) can tomato sauce
- » 1 (14.5oz) can diced tomatoes
- » 2 teaspoons oregano
- » 2 teaspoons sea salt
- » 1 teaspoon black pepper
- » 1 teaspoon cumin
- » 1 teaspoon chili powder
- » 1 teaspoon garlic powder
- » 4 cups cauliflower "rice" (see recipe on page 276)
- » 2 cups black beans, cooked and drained
- » 2 tomatoes, chopped
- » 2 avocados, sliced
- » 2 handfuls of fresh cilantro, diced
- » 2 fresh limes

Instructions

1. Combine chicken, onion, garlic, tomato sauce, diced tomatoes, and spices in a slow cooker.

2. Cook for 4 hours or until chicken is thoroughly cooked and easily pulls apart.

3. Shred or pull apart chicken with a fork.

4. On each plate, arrange chicken, cauliflower "rice," and black beans.

5. Top with tomatoes, avocado, and cilantro.

6. Squeeze lime juice over each plate and serve.

CHICKEN CURRY SALAD

Makes 4 servings

- » 1 pound chicken, cooked and shredded
- » 1 cup celery, diced
- » ½ red onion, diced
- » 1 cup green apple, diced
- » ½ cup chopped walnuts (or other nut)
- » 1 cup homemade mayonnaise (see recipe on page 229)
- » 1 tablespoon curry powder
- » ½ teaspoon sea salt

Instructions

1. Blend mayonnaise, curry powder, and sea salt.
2. Combine remaining ingredients in a large bowl.
3. Stir in dressing and chill or serve immediately.

CHICKEN FENNEL STIR FRY

Makes 4 servings

- » 2 tablespoons unrefined coconut oil
- » 1 onion, diced
- » 2 cloves garlic, minced
- » 1 fennel bulb, diced (stems optional)
- » 1-2 pounds chicken, cooked and cubed
- » 2 (14.5oz) cans diced tomatoes
- » Sea salt, to taste
- » Black pepper, to taste

Instructions

1. Heat coconut oil a large skillet on medium heat.
2. Add onion, garlic, and fennel.
3. Sauté 2-3 minutes until fennel is softened.
4. Add remaining ingredients and season to taste.
5. Serve over brown rice, quinoa, or zucchini noodles.

CHICKEN ITALIANO SALAD

Makes 4 servings

- » 2 large parsnips, cubed
- » 1 tablespoon unrefined coconut oil
- » ½ teaspoon sea salt
- » 1 red onion, sliced
- » 1 tablespoon olive oil
- » ½ teaspoon sea salt
- » ½ teaspoon Italian seasoning
- » 8 cups dark leafy mixed greens
- » 2 large boneless, skinless chicken breasts, cooked and cubed
- » 1 cup canned artichoke hearts, sliced
- » 2 cups cherry tomatoes
- » 1 cup walnuts, chopped
- » ½ cup extra virgin olive oil
- » ½ cup raw apple cider vinegar or lemon juice
- » 1 tablespoon Italian seasoning
- » ½ teaspoon powdered stevia (I recommend Stevita Supreme or SweetLeaf brand)
- » ½ teaspoon sea salt
- » ½ teaspoon black pepper

Instructions

1. Preheat oven to 400 degrees.
2. Coat parsnips with coconut oil and sea salt.

3. Place in a glass baking dish and bake for 25-35 minutes or until soft.

4. Heat a medium skillet on medium low heat.

5. Add red onion, olive oil, sea salt, and Italian seasoning.

6. Sauté onions until just slightly tender. Set aside.

7. Arrange dark leafy mixed greens on plates.

8. Top with chicken, red onion, parsnips, artichokes, cherry tomatoes and walnuts.

9. In a blender, mix remaining ingredients.

10. Pour dressing over salad.

GRILLED FENNEL CHICKEN SALAD

Makes 4 servings

- » 1-2 pounds chicken breasts, sliced into fingers
- » 1 teaspoon sea salt (divided)
- » 1 teaspoon black pepper (divided)
- » 2 tablespoon lemon zest (divided)
- » 1 fennel bulb, quartered
- » 1 yellow pepper, sliced
- » 1 orange pepper, sliced
- » 1 tablespoon extra virgin olive oil
- » 8 cups romaine lettuce, rinsed and chopped
- » 2 cups cherry tomatoes
- » 2 cucumbers, sliced
- » 4 tablespoons fresh parsley, diced
- » 1 cup extra virgin olive oil
- » 4 tablespoons lemon juice or raw apple cider vinegar
- » 1 teaspoon sea salt
- » 1 teaspoon black pepper

Instructions

1. Preheat grill to 350 degrees.

2. Season the chicken fingers with ½ teaspoon salt, ½ teaspoon pepper, and 1 tablespoon lemon zest. Place chicken on grill.

3. Combine fennel, yellow and orange peppers with ½ teaspoon salt, ½ teaspoon pepper, and 1 tablespoon lemon zest. Place veggies on grill.

4. While chicken and veggies are grilling, arrange lettuce, tomatoes, and cucumbers on individual plates.

5. Blend olive oil, lemon juice or vinegar, parsley, salt and pepper in a blender.

6. When chicken and veggies are finished, arrange them on the plates.

7. Pour dressing over salads.

ONE POT CHICKEN CURRY

Makes 8 servings

- » 1-2 pounds chicken breast, cooked and cut into 1-inch pieces
- » 2 (15.5oz) cans unsweetened coconut milk
- » 1-2 large tomatoes, diced
- » 1 (6oz) can tomato paste
- » 2 cups frozen peas
- » 1 cup cashews
- » 2 small onions, chopped and sautéed
- » 2 cloves garlic, minced and sautéed
- » 2 tablespoons coconut nectar
- » 2-3 tablespoons raw apple cider vinegar or lemon juice
- » 1 tablespoon curry powder
- » 1 teaspoon onion powder
- » 1 teaspoon black pepper
- » Salt, to taste

Instructions

1. Combine all in a slow cooker and cook on high for 4 hours.

Note: You can make this in a large skillet, as well. Sauté the chicken, followed by the onions and garlic. Add all other ingredients and cook on medium heat until thickened.

ROASTED CHICKEN

Makes 8-10 servings

- » 1 whole chicken
- » 2-3 tablespoons unrefined coconut oil
- » 1 teaspoon onion powder
- » 1 teaspoon garlic powder
- » sea salt, to taste

Instructions

1. Preheat oven to 375 degrees.
2. Remove giblets and rinse chicken for several minutes.
3. Place chicken breast side down in a glass baking dish.
4. Make 4 (1-inch) slits in the skin on top of the chicken.
5. Place a pat of coconut oil inside each slit.
6. Sprinkle seasonings over the entire chicken.
7. Bake for 1 hour or until chicken reaches 180 degrees, using a meat thermometer.
8. Remove meat, keeping any extra for additional chicken dishes.
9. Place the carcass, skin, fat, joints and all oil that collected in the glass dish in a slow cooker for preparing bone broth. (See instructions on page)

SHIRATAKI PALEO STIR FRY

Makes 4 servings

- » 2-3 tablespoon unrefined coconut oil
- » 1-2 pounds chicken breast, cooked and diced
- » 2 stalks celery, diced
- » 2 carrots, julienned
- » 1 onion, diced
- » 2 cloves garlic, diced
- » 1 wedge green cabbage, diced
- » 1 green pepper, diced
- » 2-3 tablespoons Braggs liquid aminos or coconut aminos
- » Sea salt, to taste
- » 1-inch slice of fresh ginger, minced
- » 1 teaspoon garlic powder
- » 1 cup pepitas (pumpkin seeds)
- » ½ cup sliced almonds
- » Shirataki noodles, to top
- » Romaine lettuce (optional)

Instructions

1. Heat coconut oil in a large skillet.
2. Lightly stir fry the chicken, celery, carrots, onion, garlic, cabbage, and green pepper.
3. Season the vegetables with aminos, sea salt, ginger, and garlic powder.
4. Add pepitas and almonds.
5. Serve on a bed of romaine lettuce and top with shirataki noodles (optional).

SPICY CHICKEN SOUP (SLOW COOKER)

Makes 12 servings

- » 2 tablespoons unrefined coconut oil
- » 1 onion, diced
- » 5 cloves garlic, minced
- » 1 green bell pepper, diced
- » 2 quarts bone broth
- » 6 cups chicken, cooked and cubed or shredded
- » 1 (16oz) jar sugar-free salsa
- » 3 (14.5oz) cans diced tomatoes
- » 1 (14.5oz) can tomato sauce
- » 2 (15.5oz) cans kidney beans or sugar-free chili beans
- » 2 tablespoons chili powder
- » 2 tablespoons dried parsley
- » 1 tablespoon onion powder
- » 1 teaspoon garlic powder
- » 1 teaspoon black pepper
- » ½ teaspoon sea salt

Instructions

1. Heat coconut oil in a medium skillet.
2. Lightly sauté onion, garlic, and green pepper. Place in slow cooker.
3. Add all remaining ingredients to slow cooker.
4. Cook for 4-6 hours.

WARM CHICKEN SUGAR SNAP PEA SALAD

Makes 4 servings

- » 4 tablespoons unrefined coconut oil
- » 2 cups chicken, cooked and shredded
- » 2 cups sugar snap peas
- » ½ cup black beans
- » ½ cup black olives
- » ½ cup green onions
- » 1 teaspoon creole seasoning
- » 8 cups romaine lettuce, washed and chopped
- » 4 tablespoons extra virgin olive oil

Instructions

1. Heat coconut oil in a large skillet.
2. Add chicken and sugar snap peas, and sauté for 2 minutes.
3. Add beans, olives, onions and seasoning, and continue cooking until peas are soft.
4. Serve on a bed of lettuce and drizzle olive oil on top.

FISH & SEAFOOD RECIPES

ALMOND CRUSTED WHITE FISH

Makes 4 servings

- » 4 fillets white fish (flounder, cod, trout, tilapia, etc.)
- » 1 egg
- » ¼ teaspoon sea salt
- » ¼ teaspoon black pepper
- » 1 cup ground almonds (or almond meal)
- » ¼ cup coconut flour
- » 1 teaspoon lemon zest
- » 2 tablespoons coconut oil or clarified butter

Instructions

1. Preheat oven to hi broil.
2. Whisk egg, salt, and pepper.
3. Combine almonds, coconut flour, and lemon zest in a shallow bowl.
4. Dip each fillet in egg mixture.
5. Press each side of the fillet into the almond mixture.
6. Place fillets in a glass baking dish.
7. Place a pat of coconut oil or clarified butter on top of each fillet.
8. Broil for 3-5 minutes or until fillet is done.

Note: If you have extra time, you can "fry" the fillets in a skillet with coconut oil. Any type of nut will work for this recipe. It is helpful to make a larger batch of the almond mixture and store in the freezer for future meals.

BASIC GRILLED SALMON

Makes 4 servings

- » 4 salmon fillets
- » 4 tablespoons clarified butter or coconut oil
- » ½ red onion, sliced
- » 3 cloves garlic, minced
- » 2 teaspoons dried dill weed
- » 2 teaspoons sea salt
- » 1 teaspoon onion powder
- » 1 teaspoon garlic powder
- » ½ teaspoon paprika
- » 1 lemon

Instructions

1. Turn oven on hi broil.
2. Arrange salmon fillets in a glass baking dish.
3. Spread coconut oil over each fillet.
4. Arrange garlic and onion over each fillet.
5. Sprinkle seasonings over all fillets.
6. Squeeze lemon juice over fillets.
7. Broil for 7-8 minutes.

SALMON PATTIES

Makes 5 patties

- » 2 tablespoons unrefined coconut oil
- » 1 (15oz) can wild Alaskan salmon
- » 3 eggs
- » ¼ cup coconut flour
- » ½ cup spinach, kale or Swiss chard, finely diced
- » ½ tablespoon dried parsley or 1 tablespoon fresh parsley, diced
- » ½ teaspoon sea salt
- » ½ teaspoon pepper
- » 1 teaspoon onion powder
- » 1 teaspoon garlic powder

Instructions

1. Heat coconut oil in a large skillet on medium heat.
2. Combine remaining ingredients in a medium-sized bowl.
3. Form patties and cook for 5 to 8 minutes on each side.

SALMON TACO BOWLS

Makes 4 servings

- » 2 tablespoons unrefined coconut oil
- » 4 wild-caught Alaskan salmon fillets
- » ½ teaspoon sea salt
- » ½ teaspoon black pepper
- » ½ teaspoon chili powder
- » 4 cups mixed greens
- » 3 cups cauliflower "rice" (see recipe on page 276)
- » 1 avocado, sliced
- » 1 mango, sliced
- » 1 ½ cup black beans, cooked
- » 4 tablespoons fresh cilantro, diced
- » 4 tablespoons sesame seeds

Instructions

1. Heat coconut oil in a large skillet on medium heat.
2. Add salmon fillets to skillet and season with salt, pepper, and chili powder.
3. Cover and let cook until salmon flakes with a fork.
4. Arrange mixed greens on plates.
5. Top with cauliflower "rice," avocado, mango, black beans, and salmon.
6. Sprinkle cilantro and sesame seeds on top.

SESAME ORANGE SALMON

Makes 4 servings

- » 4 wild-caught Alaskan salmon fillets

For the marinade:

- » ¼ cup unrefined coconut oil
- » 2 tablespoons sesame seed oil
- » 2 tablespoons raw apple cider vinegar
- » ½ teaspoon powdered stevia (I recommend Stevita Supreme or SweetLeaf brand)
- » 2 tablespoons coconut aminos
- » 2 cloves garlic, minced
- » 1 teaspoon dried ginger

For the glaze:

- » ½ cup unrefined coconut oil
- » 2 teaspoons powdered stevia
- » 2 teaspoons sesame oil
- » 1 teaspoons coconut aminos
- » 1 teaspoon dried ginger
- » Juice of 1/2 orange (or 5 drops of food-grade orange oil)
- » ½ teaspoon sea salt
- » ¼ teaspoon black pepper

Instructions

1. In a small bowl, combine all ingredients for the marinade.

2. Place salmon in a glass baking dish and pour marinade over fillets.

3. Let fillets marinate for 20 minutes in the refrigerator.

4. In a small bowl, combine all ingredients for the glaze. Set aside.

5. Preheat oven to hi broil.

6. Discard marinade from glass baking dish, but keep salmon in the dish.

7. Broil salmon for 10 minutes or until it flakes with a fork.

8. Pour glaze over salmon.

Note: Serve salmon over sautéed shredded cabbage and pour glaze over entire dish.

TUNA OR SALMON SALAD

Makes 2 servings

- » 1 (5oz) can light tuna or wild pink salmon, drained
- » 3 tablespoons homemade mayonnaise (see recipe on page 229)
- » 1 sprig green onion, chopped
- » 1 clove garlic, minced
- » ½ teaspoon turmeric
- » ½ teaspoon dried dill weed
- » 1 teaspoon lemon juice

Instructions

1. Mix all ingredients together in a bowl.
2. Serve over lettuce, or wrapped in a cabbage or lettuce leaf, or with celery sticks.

Note: To make a spicy version, omit the dill and add ½ teaspoon cayenne pepper and a splash of liquid smoke or sriracha.

BEEF RECIPES

ASIAN MEATBALLS

Makes 4 servings

- » 1 pound grass-fed beef
- » 2 eggs, beaten
- » 2 tablespoons green onions, chopped
- » 1 tablespoon Braggs coconut aminos
- » 1 teaspoon ginger
- » 1 clove garlic, crushed
- » ¼ cup bone broth
- » ¼ cup unrefined coconut oil
- » ¼ coconut aminos
- » 1 teaspoon powdered stevia (I recommend Stevita Supreme or SweetLeaf brand)
- » 2 tablespoons green onions, chopped
- » 2 teaspoons freshly grated ginger
- » 1 clove garlic, minced

Instructions

1. Preheat oven to 400 degrees.
2. In a large bowl, combine beef, eggs, green onions, aminos, ginger, and garlic.

3. Form 1 to 2-inch balls and arrange in a glass baking dish.

4. Bake for 20 minutes or until browned.

5. In a medium-sized saucepan, combine remaining ingredients.

6. Simmer for 10 minutes.

7. Turn off heat and let cool to thicken.

8. Pour sauce over meatballs.

MEXICAN TACO SALAD

Makes 4 servings

- » 1 pound grass-fed ground beef
- » 1 teaspoon chili powder
- » ½ teaspoon onion powder
- » ½ teaspoon garlic powder
- » ½ teaspoon oregano
- » ½ teaspoon sea salt
- » 2 tablespoons unrefined coconut oil
- » 1 onion
- » 2 green bell peppers
- » 3 cloves garlic, minced
- » ½ teaspoon sea salt
- » ½ teaspoon chili powder
- » 8 cups mixed greens
- » 2 cups black beans, cooked and drained
- » 2 tomatoes, diced
- » 2 avocados, sliced
- » ½ cup sugar-free salsa
- » Creamy avocado dressing (see recipe on page 223)

Instructions

1. Heat a medium skillet on medium heat.
2. Add ground beef and spices. Brown the beef.

3. In another medium skillet, heat coconut oil on medium heat.

4. Lightly sauté onion, garlic and green pepper.

5. Add salt and chili powder.

6. Place a bed of mixed lettuce on each plate.

7. Arrange meat, beans, onion and peppers, tomatoes and avocado on the lettuce.

8. Top with salsa and creamy avocado dressing.

PALEO HOBO DINNER

Makes 4 servings

» 1 pound grass-fed beef

» 1 teaspoon chili powder or chipotle powder

» ½ teaspoon garlic powder

» ½ teaspoon onion powder

» ½ teaspoon salt

» ½ teaspoon oregano

» ½ teaspoon basil

» 1 tablespoon unrefined coconut oil

» 1 onion, roughly chopped

» 8 carrots, roughly chopped

» 1 head cauliflower, steamed and roughly chopped

» 1 (12oz) package kelp noodles (optional)

Instructions

1. Brown the beef in a medium skillet, on medium heat.

2. Add all seasonings and ¼ cup water, if meat is dry.

3. Turn off heat and set meat aside.

4. In a large skillet, sauté carrot and onion in coconut oil, on medium heat.

5. On a plate, layer cauliflower, kelp noodles, carrot/onion mixture and beef.

Note: Hobos can be precooked and preassembled in aluminum foil, and placed on a grill or campfire to reheat.

QUICK ONE POT ROAST

Makes 4-6 servings

- » 1-3 to 5-pound chuck roast
- » 1 onion, sliced
- » 4 carrots, roughly sliced
- » 3 stalks celery, roughly sliced
- » 2 sweet potatoes, cubed
- » 4 cups bone broth
- » 4 tablespoons raw apple cider vinegar
- » 1 teaspoon sea salt
- » 1 teaspoon garlic powder
- » 1 teaspoon onion powder
- » 1 teaspoon oregano
- » 1 teaspoon basil

Instructions

1. Place all ingredients in a slow cooker.
2. Cook for 4-6 hours on high.

Note: For a heartier meal, add additional vegetables such green beans, peas, zucchini, squash, parsnips, turnips, etc.

ROBUST CHILI (SLOW COOKER)

Makes 10-12 servings

- » 2 tablespoons unrefined coconut oil or bacon fat
- » 1 large onion, diced
- » 4 stalks organic celery, diced
- » 4 cloves garlic, minced
- » 2 pounds grass-fed ground beef
- » 1 quart bone broth
- » 3 (14.5oz) cans diced tomatoes
- » 1 (15oz) can tomato sauce
- » 2 (15.5oz) cans kidney or sugar-free chili beans, rinsed and drained
- » 1 tablespoon chili powder
- » 1 teaspoon basil
- » 1 teaspoon oregano
- » 1 teaspoon cumin
- » 1 teaspoon onion powder
- » 1 teaspoon garlic powder
- » 1 teaspoon sea salt
- » 1/2 teaspoon black pepper

Instructions

1. Heat coconut oil or bacon fat in a medium skillet on medium heat.

2. Add onion, celery, and garlic and sauté for 3-4 minutes. Set aside.

3. Brown the ground beef in another medium skillet on medium heat.

4. In a slow cooker, add sautéed vegetables, ground beef, and remaining ingredients.

5. Add more broth, if needed.

6. Cook on high for 4-6 hours.

Note: I often add shredded kale, fresh cilantro or parsley, or diced green beans to increase the amount of vegetables.

VEGETABLE RECIPES

BASIC COLESLAW

Makes 4 servings

- » ¼ head green cabbage, diced
- » ¼ head purple cabbage, diced
- » 1 cup shredded carrots
- » 2 tablespoons raw apple cider vinegar or lemon juice
- » ¼ teaspoon sea salt
- » ¼ teaspoon black pepper
- » ¼ teaspoon dry mustard
- » ¼ teaspoon celery seed
- » ½ teaspoon garlic powder
- » 1/3 cup homemade mayonnaise (see recipe on page 229)

Instructions

1. Combine cabbage and carrot in a large bowl.
2. Blend remaining ingredients in a blender or using a whisk.
3. Pour dressing over the cabbage and combine well.
4. Chill in refrigerator.
5. Store in the refrigerator for up to 5 days.

Note: You can add additional diced veggies for variety.

CAULIFLOWER "MASHED POTATOES"

Makes 4 servings

- » 1 head cauliflower, roughly chopped
- » ½ teaspoon sea salt
- » ½ teaspoon black pepper
- » ½ teaspoon onion powder
- » ½ teaspoon garlic powder
- » ½ to 1 cup canned unsweetened coconut milk

Instructions

1. Steam cauliflower until softened.
2. Place cauliflower and remaining ingredients in a blender or food processor.
3. Blend until mixed, adding more coconut milk, if necessary.

CAULIFLOWER "RICE"

Makes 4 servings

» 1 head cauliflower, chopped into large pieces

» 1-2 tablespoons unrefined coconut oil or clarified butter

» sea salt, to taste

» black pepper, to taste

Instructions

1. Heat oil in a medium sized skillet on medium heat.

2. Using either a box grinder with larger holes or a food processor, grind cauliflower into small rice-sized pieces.

3. Add cauliflower to skillet and cook until softened.

4. Season with salt and pepper.

Note: Various seasonings can be added to this recipe so the "rice" compliments your dish, including: oregano, basil, chili pepper, chipotle seasoning, curry, turmeric, cumin, onion and garlic powder.

CRUCIFEROUS COCKTAIL SALAD

Makes 4 servings

» 2 small heads of broccoli, lightly steamed and chopped

» 2 stems of fresh kale, chopped

» 1 cup green cabbage, shredded

» 1 red pepper, diced

» ½ cup sunflower seeds

» ½ cup red onions, diced

» ½ cup homemade mayonnaise (see recipe on page 229)

» ¼ cup avocado oil

» 2 green apples, cored

» 2-3 tablespoons raw, apple cider vinegar or lemon juice

Instructions

1. Combine broccoli, kale, cabbage, red pepper, and red onions in a large bowl.

2. Blend mayonnaise, oil, apples, and vinegar in a blender until well combined.

3. Pour dressing over the vegetables and serve.

DETOX GREEN SOUP

Makes 4 servings

- » 2 teaspoons unrefined coconut oil
- » 2 cloves of garlic, minced
- » ¼ onion, diced
- » 1 inch of fresh ginger, peeled and chopped
- » 4 cups fresh broccoli, roughly chopped
- » 1/2 pound of fresh spinach leaves
- » 3 parsnips, peeled and chopped
- » 2 stalks celery, chopped
- » A handful of fresh parsley, roughly chopped
- » Fresh water or bone broth, as needed
- » 1 teaspoon sea salt
- » ½ teaspoon black pepper
- » ½ teaspoon turmeric
- » 1 tablespoon lemon or lime juice
- » 1 (15.5oz) can unsweetened coconut milk

Instructions

1. In a large stock pan, heat coconut oil on medium heat.
2. Add garlic, onion, and ginger. Lightly sauté.
3. Add broccoli, spinach, parsnips, celery and parsley.
4. Add enough water or broth to cover all the vegetables.
5. Bring to a simmer and cook for 20-25 minutes.

6. Add sea salt, black pepper, turmeric, and lemon juice.

7. Using a blender, blend the soup in batches until it is just slightly chunky.

8. Add coconut milk and heat through.

Note: Make a double batch and freeze extras.

MARINATED VEGETABLE SALAD

Makes 1-2 servings

- » ¼ cup extra virgin olive oil
- » 1 tablespoon lemon juice
- » pinch of sea salt
- » pinch of black pepper
- » ½ teaspoon Italian seasoning
- » ¼ teaspoon turmeric (optional, but very anti-inflammatory)
- » 2-3 cups mixed vegetables, roughly chopped (zucchini, tomato, carrots, beets, summer squash, celery, cucumber, broccoli, cauliflower, cabbage, etc.)
- » ½ cup beans, cooked and drained (optional)
- » 1-2 tablespoons nuts or seeds

Instructions

1. Combine olive oil, lemon juice and seasonings in a pint-sized glass mason jar.
2. Add all vegetables, placing firmer vegetables on the bottom and softer vegetables near the top.
3. Add beans, nuts or seeds.
4. Place lid on the jar and refrigerate until ready to serve.
5. Shake up the jar before enjoying.

Note: Several jars can be premade and stored in the refrigerator for 4-5 days. For more variation, you can add cooked chicken and grains. You can adjust the amount of dressing and add different spices.

REFRESHING POWER GREEN SALAD

Makes 4 servings

- » 8 cups power greens (spinach, kale, swiss chard)
- » 2 cucumbers, sliced
- » 2 green apples, sliced
- » 1 cup chopped pecans or walnuts
- » 1 cup extra virgin olive oil
- » 1/3 cup preservative-free lime juice
- » ½ teaspoon sea salt
- » 2 tablespoons fresh basil, or 2 teaspoons dried basil
- » ½ teaspoon powdered stevia (I recommend Stevita Supreme or SweetLeaf brand)

Instructions

1. Toss power greens, cucumber, apples, and nuts together.
2. Blend remaining ingredients.
3. Pour dressing over salad.

SWEET CURRIED BROCCOLI SALAD

Makes 4 servings

» 1 head broccoli, roughly chopped

» ½ cup red onion, diced

» ½ cup sunflower seeds

» 1 cup green apple, diced

» 1 green bell pepper, diced

» ¾ cup homemade mayonnaise (see recipe on page 229)

» 1 tablespoon lemon juice

» 2 tablespoons raw apple cider vinegar

» 1 teaspoon powdered stevia (I recommend Stevita Supreme or SweetLeaf brand)

» 1 tablespoon curry powder

Instructions

1. In a large bowl, combine broccoli, onion, seeds, apple, and green pepper.

2. In a small bowl, whisk remaining ingredients to make a dressing.

3. Combine salad and dressing.

4. Chill for at least 2 hours or overnight.

SWEET FENNEL CABBAGE SALAD

Makes 4 servings

- » ½ head of cabbage, shredded
- » 1 red pepper, diced
- » 1 green apple, diced
- » 1 (15.5oz) can unsweetened coconut milk
- » juice of ½ lemon, squeezed
- » 20 drops of clear stevia (I recommend SweetLeaf brand)
- » ½ teaspoon nutmeg
- » ½ teaspoon cinnamon
- » ½ teaspoon sea salt
- » ½ cup fresh fennel tops

Instructions

1. Combine cabbage, red pepper, and green apple in a large bowl.
2. Place remaining ingredients in a blender and mix well.
3. Pour dressing over cabbage and toss.

TROPICAL CABBAGE SALAD

Makes 4 servings

- » ½ head green cabbage, shredded
- » ¼ head purple cabbage, shredded
- » 2 stalks celery, diced
- » 1 cup berries
- » 1-2 kiwi, sliced
- » 1 cup sunflower or pumpkin seeds
- » 1 avocado
- » 1 cup canned unsweetened coconut milk
- » 2 tablespoons coconut butter
- » ¼ cup preservative-free lime juice
- » 1 teaspoon pure vanilla extract
- » ½ teaspoon powdered stevia, or more to taste (I recommend Stevita Supreme or SweetLeaf brand)
- » 1 tablespoon lemon zest

Instructions

1. Combine cabbage, celery, berries, kiwi, and seeds in a large bowl.
2. Mix all remaining ingredients in a blender.
3. Toss dressing with the cabbage salad until well coated.

VEGETABLE "FRIES"

Makes 4 servings

- » 8 cups of any of the following: sweet potatoes, carrots, parsnip, jicama, beets, sliced into thin "sticks"
- » ½ cup melted unrefined coconut oil
- » 1 teaspoon sea salt
- » 1 tablespoon mixed seasonings of your choice: cinnamon, nutmeg, smoked paprika, basil, onion powder, garlic powder, turmeric, ginger, curry, etc.

Instructions

1. Preheat oven to 400 degrees.
2. Place vegetable sticks in a large gallon-sized bag.
3. Pour melted (but not hot!) oil over the vegetables.
4. Add salt and desired seasonings.
5. Shake bag until vegetables are well coated.
6. Spread veggie sticks on a baking sheet in a single layer.
7. Bake for 20 to 25 minutes or until slightly crispy.

WARM CHILI CABBAGE SLAW

Makes 4 servings

- » 2-3 tablespoons unrefined coconut oil
- » 5-6 cups green cabbage, shredded
- » 2 large green apples, diced
- » 1 green pepper, sliced
- » 1 handful fresh cilantro, chopped
- » 3/4 cup pumpkin seeds
- » 2 (15.5oz) cans no-sugar chili beans, drained, or self-prepared pinto beans
- » Sea salt, to taste

Instructions

1. Heat coconut oil in a large skillet over medium heat.
2. Add all ingredients to the skillet and sauté lightly.
3. Serve warm.

ZUCCHINI NOODLES

Makes 2 servings

» 1 large zucchini

Instructions

There are 2 ways to shape zucchini into noodles:

1. Use a spiralizer to make noodles from the whole zucchini, or

2. Use a vegetable peeler to peel zucchini into slices. Use a knife to slice peels lengthwise into noodle shapes.

Zucchini noodles can be used raw, or you can cook them to soften.

Instructions to cook zucchini noodles

1. Heat 1-2 teaspoons of olive oil or clarified butter in a skillet, over medium heat.

2. Stir in zucchini noodles and cook for 1-2 minutes.

3. Add 2 tablespoons of water and cook until tender.

4. Drain excess liquid.

GRAIN/LEGUME/BEAN RECIPES

ALMOND QUICK BREAD

Makes 1 loaf

- » 1 ½ cups fine-ground almond flour or almond meal
- » ¾ cup tapioca starch
- » ¼ cup ground flaxseed
- » ½ teaspoon sea salt
- » ½ teaspoon baking soda
- » 4 eggs
- » 1 teaspoon powdered stevia (I recommend Stevita Supreme or SweetLeaf brand)
- » 1 teaspoon lemon juice

Instructions

1. Preheat oven to 350 degrees.
2. Grease a loaf pan with coconut oil and line the bottom with a piece of parchment paper.
3. Combine almond flour, tapioca, flaxseed, salt, and baking soda in a medium bowl.
4. Whisk eggs for 3 to 5 minutes, until frothy.
5. Add stevia and lemon juice into the eggs.
6. Mix the dry ingredients into the egg mixture.

7. Pour into the loaf pans.

8. Bake for 30 to 35 minutes or until a toothpick comes out clean.

9. Allow to cool before slicing.

Note: Tapioca starch is not generally recommended for gut healing, but in the context of this recipe, its effects are countered with the high fat content of almonds and flax. However, I would only suggest consuming 1 piece of this "bread" each day, if you are healing your gut. Extra can be stored in the freezer.

BAKED BROWN RICE OR QUINOA

Makes 4 servings

- » 3 cups bone broth
- » 1 cup brown rice, or 1½ cups quinoa
- » 1 teaspoon sea salt
- » 1 teaspoon onion powder or flakes
- » 1 teaspoon garlic powder or fresh minced garlic
- » 1 teaspoon basil
- » 1 teaspoon oregano
- » ½ teaspoon black pepper

Instructions

1. Preheat oven to 350 degrees.
2. Combine all ingredients in an oven-safe ceramic or glass baking dish.
3. Bake for 1 ½ hours for brown rice or 50 minutes for quinoa, or until all liquid is absorbed.
4. Fluff with a fork.

Note: If you have an Instant Pot or pressure cooker, you can use this same recipe, but adjust the liquid according to your device's instruction manual.

QUINOA BEAN BERRY SALAD

Makes 4 servings

» 2 cups quinoa (see Baked Quinoa recipe on page 290)

» 2 cups garbanzo beans (chickpeas), cooked and drained

» 2 cups fresh berries (any assortment of blueberries, blackberries, raspberries)

» 2 cups nuts or seeds (any assortment of pumpkin seeds, sliced almonds, cashews, pecans, walnuts, sunflower seeds)

» 1 handful fresh dill, diced

» 1 handful fresh parsley, diced

» 1 cup extra virgin olive oil or avocado oil

» ½ cup raw apple cider vinegar, or lemon juice

» ½ teaspoon black pepper

» ½ teaspoon sea salt

» ½ teaspoon powdered stevia, or more to taste (I recommend Stevita Supreme or SweetLeaf brand)

» 8 cups spinach

Instructions

1. Combine quinoa, beans, berries, nuts or seeds, dill and parsley in a large bowl.

2. Mix olive oil, vinegar or lemon juice, black pepper, salt, and stevia in a blender.

3. Pour dressing over the salad and toss.

4. Serve on a bed of spinach.

GUT-FRIENDLY DESSERTS

Frozen Almond Butter Cups

Makes 12 cups

Chocolate Coating

- » 2/3 cup unsweetened raw cacao powder
- » 1/3 cup unrefined coconut oil
- » 1 tablespoon unsulfured molasses
- » 1 teaspoon pure vanilla extract
- » 1 pinch powdered stevia (I recommend Stevita Supreme or SweetLeaf brand)

Filling

- » ½ cup canned 100% pumpkin puree
- » ½ cup natural almond butter
- » 1 pear, blended with 3 tablespoons avocado oil
- » ½ teaspoon cinnamon
- » ¼ teaspoon nutmeg
- » ¼ teaspoon sea salt

Instructions

1. Line 12 muffin cups with paper liners.

2. Combine all ingredients for the chocolate coating in a small saucepan.

3. Heat all ingredients on low heat, until melted.

4. Remove from heat.

5. Combine all ingredients for the filling in a small bowl and mix well.

6. Spoon 2 tablespoons of the chocolate into each muffin cup.

7. Spoon the filling into each cup, dividing between all cups.

8. Pour the remaining chocolate over the filling, dividing between all cups.

9. Using a toothpick, make 3-4 gentle swirls in each cup.

10. Freeze the cups for 2 to 3 hours.

11. Remove liners and serve immediately.

FUDGY CHOCOLATE BROWNIES

Makes 12 brownies

» 1 ½ cups sugar-free dark chocolate chips (i.e. Lily's Premium Baking Chips)

» 1 (15.5oz) can black beans, rinsed and drained

» ¼ cup raw cacao powder

» 2 eggs, beaten

» 1/3 cup unrefined coconut oil, melted

» ¼ teaspoon cinnamon

» 2 teaspoons pure vanilla extract

» ¼ teaspoon sea salt

» ½ teaspoon baking powder

» 1 teaspoon organic instant coffee (optional)

» 1 tablespoon powdered stevia (I recommend Stevita Supreme or SweetLeaf brand)

Instructions

1. Preheat oven to 350 degrees.

2. Combine all ingredients in a strong blender or food processor and blend until smooth.

3. Line an 8x8 glass baking dish with parchment paper.

4. Pour batter into glass baking dish and spread with a spatula.

5. Bake for 30 minutes or until firm.

6. Cool before cutting into squares.

HOT CHOCOLATE

Makes 4 small servings

» 1 (15.5oz) can unsweetened coconut milk

» 2 cups filtered water

» 2 teaspoons pure vanilla extract

» 1 teaspoon stevia (I recommend Stevita Supreme or SweetLeaf brand)

» 2 tablespoons raw cacao powder

» pinch of cinnamon

» 1 teaspoon instant organic coffee (optional, but enhances the flavor)

Instructions

1. Combine all ingredients in a medium-sized saucepan.

2. Heat on medium heat until warm.

HEALTHY "SODA"

Makes 1 serving

» 12 ounces carbonated mineral water (i.e. Perrier), chilled

» 10 drops of SweetLeaf flavored liquid stevia

Instructions

1. Add stevia drops to mineral water and gently stir.

Note: To make a mock 7 Up or Sprite, add 1 tablespoon lemon juice and 1 tablespoon preservative-free lime juice.

LIME OR DARK CHOCOLATE AVOCADO MOUSSE

Makes 2 servings

- » 1 avocado, seeded
- » ¼ cup preservative-free lime juice, or 2 freshly squeezed limes
- » 1 tablespoon unrefined coconut oil
- » ¼ teaspoon ground ginger
- » 12 drops liquid stevia (I recommend SweetLeaf brand)

Instructions

1. Combine all ingredients in a blender and mix well.
2. Pour into 2 individual cups.
3. Freeze for 20 to 30 minutes.

Dark Chocolate Mousse: Omit the lime juice and replace it with 3 tablespoons raw cacao powder. To enrich the chocolate flavor, add a pinch of organic instant coffee, a sprinkle of cinnamon, and a dash of salt.

NUT BUTTER FIBER COOKIES

Makes 12 cookies

» 1 ¼ cups cooked garbanzo beans, drained and rinsed

» 2/3 cup natural almond butter (or other non-peanut nut butter)

» 2 ½ teaspoons powdered stevia (I recommend Stevita Supreme or SweetLeaf brand)

» 2 teaspoons pure almond extract

» 1 teaspoon baking powder

Instructions

1. Preheat oven to 350 degrees.

2. Line a baking sheet with parchment paper.

3. Place all ingredients in a high-powered blender and blend until a stiff batter forms. You may have to scrape the sides often and push down the contents.

4. Place spoonfuls of dough onto the baking sheet and press dough down lightly with a fork dipped in water.

5. Bake for 10-12 minutes.

6. Let cool so cookies can harden.

PEPPERMINT PATTIES

Makes 8 patties

- » ½ cup unsweetened shredded coconut
- » ½ cup unrefined coconut oil
- » 20 drops liquid stevia (I recommend SweetLeaf brand)
- » 1/3 teaspoon food-grade, pure peppermint oil
- » 3 ounces sugar-free chocolate

Instructions

1. Melt coconut oil in a small saucepan on medium-low heat, but don't overheat.
2. Combine the shredded coconut, coconut oil, and stevia.
3. Once mixture is combined and cool, add peppermint oil.
4. Pour mixture into the bottom of 8 muffin trays.
5. Freeze muffin tray for 20 minutes, or until coconut mixture is solid.
6. Heat 2-3 inches of water in a medium-sized saucepan on medium heat and nestle a smaller saucepan within it.
7. Turn your heat to low and place your chocolate in the smaller saucepan to melt it, stirring continuously.
8. Remove your melted chocolate from the heat.
9. Pop out each coconut patty from the muffin tin, dip it in the melted chocolate and return it to the muffin tin. Repeat for each coconut patty.
10. Any remaining chocolate can be divided between the muffin tins by pouring it on top of the patties.
11. Refreeze for 15 minutes or until solid.
12. Keep stored in the freezer.

SHOPPING LISTS

The shopping lists accommodate the grain-free menu options and a Morning Shake on Mondays and Thursdays. Amounts are provided according to recipe serving sizes. You may need to adjust quantities based on your family's size.

Week 1

Meat, Poultry & Fish

» Whey protein powder - from raw milk, grass-fed cows, minimally processed

» 2 whole free-range chickens

» 2 pounds boneless, skinless chicken breasts (or meat from whole chickens)

» 3 to 5-pound chuck roast

» 3 pounds grass-fed ground beef

» 4 wild-caught Alaskan salmon fillets

» 1 (15oz) can wild-caught pink Alaskan salmon

» 2 dozen free-range eggs

» 1 quart bone broth

Produce

» 1 green apple

- » 3 avocados
- » 2 cups frozen berries
- » 2 heads green cabbage
- » 1 package carrots
- » 1 head cauliflower
- » 1 bunch celery
- » 1 bunch fresh cilantro
- » 2 citrus fruit (orange, tangerine, grapefruit)
- » 2 cucumbers
- » 2 fennel bulbs
- » 11 cloves garlic
- » 1 bunch kale
- » 20 cups mixed greens
- » 1 red onion
- » 4 onions
- » 1 sprig green onion
- » 1 bunch fresh parsley
- » 2 green bell peppers
- » 1 orange bell pepper
- » 1 yellow bell pepper
- » 2 sweet potatoes
- » 2 cups cherry tomatoes
- » 2 tomatoes
- » 4 medium zucchini
- » 5 cups extra veggies (for stir fry, frittata, and marinated salad)

Beans, Nuts & Seeds

- » Natural almond butter

» 2.5 cups black beans

» 2 cans kidney or sugar-free chili beans

» ¼ cup sesame seeds

» ½ cup sunflower seeds

» 1 cup walnuts

Canned/Packaged Goods

» 2 (13.5oz) cans coconut milk (I recommend Native Forest Unsweetened Organic Coconut Milk)

» 5 (14.5oz) cans organic diced tomatoes

» 1 (15oz) can organic tomato sauce

Oils, Dressings & Condiments

» Avocado oil

» Homemade mayonnaise

» Hummus

» Lemon juice

» Raw apple cider vinegar (I recommend Braggs brand)

» Sugar-free salsa

» Unrefined, cold-pressed coconut oil

Seasonings

» Basil

» Black pepper

» Chili powder

» Cinnamon

» Cumin

» Curry powder

» Dill weed

» Garlic powder

» Italian seasoning

» Onion powder

» Oregano

» Sea salt

» Turmeric

Baking Goods

» Baking soda

» ½ cup coconut flour

» ¼ cup ground flaxseed

» Powdered stevia (I recommend Stevita Supreme or SweetLeaf brand)

Week 1 Preparation: Make mayonnaise, creamy avocado dressing, sauerkraut, roast chicken (freeze meat and use carcass to make bone broth), bone broth, chicken curry salad, and marinated vegetable salad. Cut up celery sticks and veggies for snacking.

WEEK 2

Meat, Poultry & Fish

» Whey protein powder - from raw milk, grass-fed cows, minimally processed

» 1 whole free-range chicken

» 3-4 pounds boneless, skinless chicken breast (or meat from whole chickens)

» 1 pound ground pork, turkey, chicken, or beef

» 1 pound grass-fed beef

» 1 package sugar-free bacon

» 4 wild-caught Alaskan salmon fillets

» 4 fillets white fish (flounder, cod, trout, tilapia, etc.)

» 3 dozen eggs

» 1-2 quarts fresh water or bone broth

Produce

» 1 green apple

» 1 avocado

» 3 cups frozen berries

» 4 heads broccoli

» 1 head green cabbage

» 1 head purple cabbage

» 2 packages carrots

» 2 heads cauliflower

- » 1 bunch celery
- » 1 bunch fresh cilantro
- » 1 fennel bulb
- » 6 cloves garlic
- » 1 inch fresh ginger
- » 1 bunch kale
- » 1 lemon
- » 1 mango
- » 16 cups mixed greens
- » 1 red onion
- » 4 onions
- » 1 bunch green onion
- » 2 bunches fresh parsley
- » 5 parsnips
- » 2 cups frozen peas
- » 1 green bell pepper
- » 2 spaghetti squash
- » 5 sweet potatoes
- » 2 cups cherry tomatoes
- » 2 tomatoes
- » 3 medium zucchini or shirataki noodles
- » 1 zucchini
- » 5 cups extra veggies (for marinated salad)

Beans, Nuts & Seeds

- » 1 cup ground almonds (or almond meal)
- » Natural almond butter
- » 1 cup cashews

» 2 cups walnuts

» 1 ½ cup black beans, cooked

Canned/Packaged Goods

» 1 jar artichoke hearts

» 4 (15oz) cans coconut milk (I recommend Native Forest Unsweetened Organic Coconut Milk)

» 1 (15oz) can pure pumpkin puree

» 1 (6oz) can tomato paste

» 2 (14.5oz) cans diced tomatoes

» 1 (12oz) package kelp noodles (optional)

Oils, Dressings & Condiments

» Coconut butter (I recommend Artisana or MaraNatha brand)

» Coconut nectar

» Extra virgin olive oil

» Homemade mayonnaise

» Hummus

» Lemon juice

» Raw apple cider vinegar (I recommend Braggs brand)

» Unrefined, cold-pressed coconut oil

Seasonings

» Basil

» Black pepper

» Celery seed

» Chili powder

» Cinnamon

» Curry powder

» Dry mustard

» Fennel seeds

» Garlic powder

» Ginger

» Italian seasoning

» Nutmeg

» Onion powder

» Oregano

» Sage

» Sea salt

» Thyme

» Turmeric

Baking Goods

» 1 ½ cups fine-ground almond flour

» ½ cup unsweetened almond or coconut milk

» Baking powder

» Baking soda

» 2 cups coconut flour

» 1 cup unsweetened shredded coconut

» 1 cup flaxmeal

» Powdered stevia (I recommend Stevita Supreme or SweetLeaf brand)

» Pure vanilla extract

» Pure orange extract (optional)

Week 2 Preparation: Make mayonnaise, creamy avocado dressing, sauerkraut, roast chicken (freeze meat and use carcass to make bone broth), bone broth, morning glory muffins, and marinated vegetable salad. Cut up celery sticks and veggies for snacking.

WEEK 3

Meat, Poultry & Fish

» Whey protein powder - from raw milk, grass-fed cows, minimally processed

» 1 whole free-range chicken

» 2 pounds boneless, skinless chicken breasts (or meat from whole chickens)

» 1 pound ground pork, turkey, chicken, or beef

» 1 package sugar-free bacon

» 2 pounds grass-fed ground beef

» 1 (15oz) can wild Alaskan salmon

» 4 fillets white fish (flounder, cod, trout, tilapia, etc.)

» 4 dozen eggs

» 3 quarts bone broth

Produce

» 3 green apples

» 3 avocados

» 4 cups frozen berries

» 1 head broccoli

» 1 head green cabbage

» 1 head purple cabbage

» 1 package carrots

» 1 head cauliflower

» 1 bunch celery

» 1 bunch fresh cilantro

» 2 cucumbers

» 9 cloves garlic

» 1 inch fresh ginger

» 2 bunches kale

» 1-2 kiwi

» 1 lemon

» 2 fresh limes

» 8 cups mixed greens

» 2 red onions

» 5 onions

» 1 bunch green onion

» 1 bunch fresh parsley

» 2 parsnips

» 2 cups frozen peas

» 2 green bell peppers

» 8 cups power greens (spinach, kale, swiss chard)

» 2 spaghetti squash

» 2 sweet potatoes

» 2 cups cherry tomatoes

» 4 tomatoes

» 3 medium zucchini

» 4 cups extra veggies (for marinated salad and omelets)

Beans, Nuts & Seeds

» Natural almond butter

» 1 cups ground almonds (or almond meal)

» 1 cup cashews

» 1 ½ cups sunflower seeds

» 1 cup pumpkin seeds

» 2 cups walnuts

» 2 (15.5oz) cans kidney beans or sugar-free chili beans

» 2 cups black beans, cooked

Canned/Packaged Goods

» ½ cup unsweetened almond or coconut milk

» 1 jar artichoke hearts

» 4 (13.5oz) cans coconut milk (I recommend Native Forest Unsweetened Organic Coconut Milk)

» 1 (15oz) can pure pumpkin puree

» 1 (16oz) jar sugar-free salsa

» 1 (6oz) can tomato paste

» 2 (8oz) cans tomato sauce

» 4 (14.5oz) cans diced tomatoes

Oils, Dressings & Condiments

» Braggs coconut aminos

» Coconut nectar

» Extra virgin olive oil

» Homemade mayonnaise

» Hummus

» Lemon juice

» Preservative-free lime juice

» Raw apple cider vinegar (I recommend Braggs brand)

» Unrefined, cold-pressed coconut oil

Seasonings

» Basil

- » Black pepper
- » Chili powder
- » Cinnamon
- » Cumin
- » Curry powder
- » Fennel seeds
- » Garlic powder
- » Ginger
- » Italian seasoning
- » Onion powder
- » Oregano
- » Sage
- » Sea salt
- » Thyme

Baking Goods

- » 1 ½ cups fine-ground almond flour
- » ½ cup unsweetened almond or coconut milk
- » Baking soda
- » Baking powder
- » 2 cups coconut flour
- » ¼ cup flaxmeal (optional)
- » Powdered stevia (I recommend Stevita Supreme or SweetLeaf brand)
- » Pure vanilla extract

Week 3 Preparation: Make mayonnaise, creamy avocado dressing, sauerkraut, roast chicken (freeze meat and use carcass to make bone broth), bone broth, apple cinnamon muffins, and marinated vegetable salad. Cut up celery sticks and veggies for snacking.

WEEK 4

Meat, Poultry & Fish

» Whey protein powder - from raw milk, grass-fed cows, minimally processed

» 1 whole free-range chicken

» 1 pound boneless, skinless chicken breasts

» 1 pound ground pork, turkey, chicken, or beef

» 1 package sugar-free bacon

» 3 to 5 pounds chuck roast

» 3 pounds grass-fed ground beef

» 4 wild-caught Alaskan salmon fillets

» 4 fillets white fish (flounder, cod, trout, tilapia, etc.)

» 4 dozen eggs

» 3 quarts bone broth

Produce

» 2 acorn squash

» 9 green apples

» 2 avocados

» 3 cups frozen berries

» 4 heads broccoli

» 1 head green cabbage

» 2 package carrots

» 1 head cauliflower

- » 1 bunch celery
- » 2 cucumbers
- » 7 cloves garlic
- » 1 inch fresh ginger
- » 2-3 cups green beans
- » 1 bunch kale
- » 1 lemon
- » 12 cups mixed greens
- » 1 red onion
- » 4 onions
- » 1 bag oranges
- » 1 bunch fresh parsley
- » 3 parsnips
- » 2 green bell peppers
- » 1 red bell pepper
- » 10 cups power greens (spinach, kale, swiss chard)
- » 1/2 pound of fresh spinach
- » 2 tomatoes
- » 3 medium zucchini
- » 6 cups extra veggies (for stir fry and omelet)

Beans, Nuts & Seeds

- » Natural almond butter
- » 1 cup ground almonds (or almond meal)
- » 1 cup cashews
- » ½ cup sunflower seeds
- » 2 cup walnuts
- » 2 cups black beans, cooked

Canned/Packaged Goods

» 4 (13.5oz) cans coconut milk (I recommend Native Forest Unsweetened Organic Coconut Milk)

» 2 (15oz) cans pure pumpkin puree

» 1 (16oz) jar sugar-free salsa

» 1 (12 ounce) package kelp noodles (optional)

Oils, Dressings & Condiments

» Avocado oil

» Braggs coconut aminos

» Coconut butter (I recommend Artisana or MaraNatha brand)

» Extra virgin olive oil

» Homemade mayonnaise

» Hummus

» Lemon juice

» Preservative-free lime juice

» Raw apple cider vinegar (I recommend Braggs brand)

» Sesame seed oil

» Unrefined, cold-pressed coconut oil

Seasonings

» Basil

» Black pepper

» Chili powder

» Cinnamon

» Curry powder

» Fennel seeds

» Garlic powder

» Ginger

» Nutmeg

» Onion powder

» Oregano

» Sage

» Sea salt

» Thyme

» Turmeric

Baking Goods

» 1 ½ cups fine-ground almond flour

» ½ cup unsweetened almond or coconut milk

» Baking soda

» 1 ½ cups coconut flour

» 1 cup unsweetened shredded coconut

» ½ cup flaxmeal

» Powdered stevia (I recommend Stevita Supreme or SweetLeaf brand)

» Pure vanilla extract

» Pure orange extract

Week 4 Preparation: Make mayonnaise, creamy avocado dressing, sauerkraut, roast chicken (freeze meat and use carcass to make bone broth), bone broth, and chicken curry salad. Cut up celery sticks and veggies for snacking.

BEVERAGE IDEAS

- Flavored water with fresh fruit slices such as orange, lemon, lime, and berries. Add fresh mint leaves or cucumber. Sweeten with fruit-flavored liquid stevia.

- Iced, fruit-flavored herbal teas.

- Lemon-ade: water, freshly squeezed lemon, and stevia.

- Orang-ade: water, freshly squeezed orange, and stevia.

- Iced coffee with coconut milk and stevia.

- Bulletproof coffee: Blend 8 ounces strongly brewed organic coffee with 1 tablespoon coconut oil. Add whey protein powder for extra stamina and stevia to sweeten.

- "Soda" water: sparkling mineral water with flavored liquid stevia. (See recipe for Healthy "Soda.")

- Water kefir: a fizzy, probiotic drink flavored with freshly squeezed lemon, lime, orange. (See **www.bodyecology.com** for instructions on how to obtain kefir grains and make your own water kefir.)

- Coconut kefir: a probiotic drink made from either coconut water or coconut milk. (See **www.bodyecology.com** for instructions on how to obtain kefir grains and make your own coconut kefir.)

SNACK IDEAS

- Vegetables and hummus
  - Cherry tomatoes
  - Cucumber slices
  - Celery sticks
  - Baby carrots
  - Jicama sticks
  - Bell pepper slices
- Nuts (dry roasted or raw)
- Dried coconut flakes or slices
- Seaweed sheets
- Sugar-free, grass-fed or pastured jerky
- Hard-boiled or deviled eggs
- Kale "chips"
- Unsweetened, plain coconut yogurt
- Berries with coconut cream (blended coconut fat and stevia)

ONLINE SHOPPING

All the following websites offer healthy foods, natural body care products, natural household products, supplements, essential oils, and more at a discounted price.

Amazon
www.amazon.com

Vitacost
www.vitacost.com

Jet
www.jet.com

FIND A LOCAL FUNCTIONAL MEDICINE PRACTITIONER

The Institute for Functional Medicine
www.functionalmedicine.org

FIND LOCAL FARMS, CSAs, and FARMER'S MARKETS

Local Harvest
www.localharvest.org

Eat Wild
www.eatwild.com

Local Farm Markets.org
www.localfarmmarkets.org

RECOMMENDED WEBSITES

Environmental Working Group
www.ewg.org/consumer-guides
The ultimate resource for discovering toxin loads in body care products, cleaners, water, air, food and more.

The Cornucopia Institute
www.cornucopia.org
Provides scorecards and reports for the latest nutrition issues and quality food products.

SIBO Information
www.siboinfo.com
Comprehensive resource for understanding SIBO.

FODMAPs
www.ibsdiets.org/fodmap-diet/fodmap-food-list/
Complete list of foods with FODMAPs.

Glycemic Load (GL)
www.mendosa.com/gilists.htm
This provides the GL of approximately 2,400 foods, but this list may not include a lot of vegetables.

www.glycemicindex.com/
If you are searching for the GL of a specific food, this offers the most comprehensive database.

Stony Brook University Seafood Mercury Database
www.stonybrook.edu/commcms/gelfond/fish/database.html
A database of mercury levels in US commercial fish. This list combines FDA data with scientific literature for a more accurate list.

Body Ecology
www.bodyecology.com
The ultimate resource for fermentation guides and supplies.

The Candida Diet
www.thecandidadiet.com
Information and resources on Candida.

Gluten-Free Living
www.glutenfreeliving.com
A complete resource for gluten-free living.

Living Without
www.glutenfreeandmore.com
A complete resource for living with a multitude of food allergies.

Find Me Gluten Free
www.findmeglutenfree.com
Offers a free app that is useful for finding restaurants that offer gluten-free menus.

Minimalist Baker
minimalistbaker.com
Healthy recipes with 10 ingredients or less, and many are allergy friendly.

Dr. Josh Axe: Food Is Medicine
www.draxe.com
Healthy recipes, natural remedies, and articles from a functional medicine practitioner.

Dr. Jill Carnahan, Your Functional Medicine Expert®
www.jillcarnahan.com

ABOUT THE AUTHOR

Nicole Spear is a passionate teacher, lecturer, and counselor of nutrition and health. As a Certified Nutrition Specialist® professional and a Certified Functional Medicine Practitioner®, she uses an integrative, science-based approach to disease prevention and wellness. Nicole is the owner of Pure Life Health & Wellness, LLC, an independent business providing nutrition counseling to individuals and groups. She has worked with physicians, other health care providers, and clients to develop individualized nutrition and nutraceutical plans to support a variety of health concerns. Nicole has developed and taught university nutrition courses, and is an avid researcher and writer.

Contact Information

Please join Nicole's blog for more information on health conditions, nutrition, and wellness. New recipes, videos, and podcasts will be arriving soon as she expands Pure Life Health & Wellness to the online community. Nicole is accepting new clients and can work with you to restore your gut health either locally or through phone/Skype consults.

Website:
www.purelifehw.com

Email:
nicole@purelifehw.com

ENDNOTES

1. Forsythe, P., Kunze, W., & Bienenstock, J. (2016). Moody microbes or fecal phrenology: What do we know about the microbiota-gut-brain axis? *BMC Medicine, 14*: 58. http://doi.org/10.1186/s12916-016-0604-8

2. Christakos, S., Dhawan, P., Porta, A., Mady, L. J., & Seth, T. (2011). Vitamin D and intestinal calcium absorption. *Molecular and Cellular Endocrinology, 347*(1-2): 25–29. http://doi.org/10.1016/j.mce.2011.05.038

3. Peacock, M. (2010). Calcium metabolism in health and disease. *Clinical Journal of the American Society of Nephrology, 5*: S23–S30. doi: 10.2215/CJN.05910809

4. Gennari, F.J. & Weise, W.J. (2008). Acid-base disturbances in gastrointestinal disease. *Clinical Journal of the American Society of Nephrology, 3*(6): 1861-1868. doi: 10.2215/CJN.02450508

5. Zofková I. & Matucha P. (2014). New insights into the physiology of bone regulation: The role of neurohormones. *Physiological Research*, 63(4): 421-427.

6. Bindels, L.B., & Delzenne, N.M. (2013). Muscle wasting: The gut microbiota as a new therapeutic target? *International Journal of Biochemistry and Cell Biology, 45*(10): 2186-2190. doi: 10.1016/j.biocel.2013.06.021

7. Chistiakov, D. A., Bobryshev, Y. V., Kozarov, E., Sobenin, I. A., & Orekhov, A. N. (2015). Role of gut microbiota in the modulation of

atherosclerosis-associated immune response. *Frontiers in Microbiology*, *6*: 671. http://doi.org/10.3389/fmicb.2015.00671

8. Biasucci, L.M., Romito, A., Marini, M., et al. (2014). Is increased intestinal permeability associated with altered inflammatory balance and coronary artery disease? *Journal of the American College of Cardiology 63*(12_S): A181. doi: 10.1016/S0735-1097(14)60181-9

9. Ettinger, G., MacDonald, K., Reid, G., & Burton, J. P. (2014). The influence of the human microbiome and probiotics on cardiovascular health. *Gut Microbes*, *5*(6): 719–728. doi: 10.4161/19490976.2014.983775

10. Schuijt, T. J., et al. (2016). The gut microbiota plays a protective role in the host defence against pneumococcal pneumonia. *Gut*, *65*(4): 575–583. doi: 10.1136/gutjnl-2015-309728

11. Rehfeld, J.F. (2014). Gastrointestinal hormones and their targets. *Advances in Experiemental Medicine and Biology 817*: 157-175. doi: 10.1007/978-1-4939-0897-4_7.

12. Rehfeld, J.F. (2012). Beginnings: A reflection on the history of gastrointestinal endocrinology. *Regulatory Peptides 177* (Suppl:S1-5). doi: 10.1016/j.regpep.2012.05.087

13. Clark, G., et al. (2014). Minireview: Gut microbiota: The neglected

14. endocrine organ. *Molecular Endocrinology*, *28*(8): 1221-1238. doi: 10.1210/me.2014-1108

15. Vajro, P., Paolella, G., & Fasano, A. (2013). Microbiota and gut-liver axis: A mini-review on their influences on obesity and obesity related liver disease. *Journal of Pediatric Gastroenterology and Nutrition*, *56*(5): 461–468. http://doi.org/10.1097/MPG.0b013e318284abb5

16. Ilan, Y. (2012). Leaky gut and the liver: A role for bacterial translocation in nonalcoholic steatohepatitis. *World Journal of Gastroenterology 18*(21): 2609–2618. http://doi.org/10.3748/wjg.v18.i21.2609

17. Comninos, A. N., Jayasena, C. N., & Dhillo, W. S. (2014). The relationship between gut and adipose hormones, and reproduction. *Human Reproduction Update*, *20*(2): 153-174. doi: 10.1093/humupd/dmt033

18. Guo, Y., Qi, Y., Yang, X., Zhao, L., Wen, S., Liu, Y., & Tang, L. (2016). Association between polycystic ovary syndrome and gut microbiota. *PLoS ONE*, *11*(4): e0153196. http://doi.org/10.1371/journal.pone.0153196

19. Laschke M. W. & Menger M. D. (2016). The gut microbiota: A puppet master in the pathogenesis of endometriosis? *American Journal of Obstetrics and Gynecology pii*: S0002-9378(16)00336-7. doi: 10.1016/j.ajog.2016.02.036. [Epub ahead of print]

20. Gomez de Agüero, M. G., et al. (2016). The maternal microbiota drives early postnatal innate immune development. *Science, 351*(6279): 1296-302. doi: 10.1126/science.aad2571

21. Min, Y. W. & Rhee, P. L. (2015). The role of microbiota on the gut immunology. *Clinical Therapeutics, 37*(5): 968-75. doi: 10.1016/j.clinthera.2015.03.009.

22. Antifungal agents for common paediatric infections. (2008). *The Canadian Journal of Infectious Diseases & Medical Microbiology, 19*(1): 15–18.

23. Wu, H. J., & Wu, E. (2012). The role of gut microbiota in immune homeostasis and autoimmunity. *Gut Microbes, 3*(1): 4–14. http://doi.org/10.4161/gmic.19320

24. Hakansson, A., & Molin, G. (2011). Gut microbiota and inflammation. *Nutrients, 3*(6): 637–682. http://doi.org/10.3390/nu3060637

25. Michielan, A., & D'Incà, R. (2015). Intestinal Permeability in Inflammatory Bowel Disease: Pathogenesis, Clinical Evaluation, and Therapy of Leaky Gut. *Mediators of Inflammation, 2015*: 628157. http://doi.org/10.1155/2015/628157

26. Putignani, L., et al. (2016). Gut microbiota dysbiosis as risk and premorbid factors of IBD and IBS along the childhood-adulthood transition. *Inflammatory Bowel Diseases, 22*(2): 487-504. doi: 10.1097/MIB.0000000000000602

27. Li, J. J., & Chen, J. L. (2005). Inflammation may be a bridge connecting hypertension and atherosclerosis. *Medical Hypotheses, 64*(5): 925-9.

28. Shacter, E. & Weitzman, S.A. (2002). Chronic inflammation and cancer. Oncology. Retrieved from http://www.cancernetwork.com/review-article/chronic-inflammation-and-cancer

29. Hasler, W. L. (2008). Gastroparesis: Current concepts and considerations. *The Medscape Journal of Medicine, 10*(1): 16.

30. Environmental Working Group. (2005). Body Burden: The Pollution in Newborns. Retrieved from http://www.ewg.org/research/body-burden-pollution-newborns

31. Swanson, H. I. (2015). Drug metabolism by the host and gut microbiota: A partnership or rivalry? *Drug Metabolism and Disposition, 43*(10): 1499–1504. http://doi.org/10.1124/dmd.115.065714

32. Flórez, A. B., Sierra, M., Ruas-Madiedo, P., & Mayo, B. (2016). Susceptibility of lactic acid bacteria, bifidobacteria and other bacteria of intestinal origin to chemotherapeutic agents. *International Journal of Antimicrobial Agents, 48*(5): 547-550. doi:10.1016/j.ijantimicag.2016.07.011

33. Otani, K., et al. (2017). Microbiota Plays a Key Role in Non-Steroidal Anti-Inflammatory Drug-Induced Small Intestinal Damage. *Digestion, 95*(1), 22-28. doi:10.1159/000452356

34. Chassaing, B., et al. (2015). Dietary emulsifiers impact the mouse gut microbiota promoting colitis and metabolic syndrome. *Nature, 519*(7541): 92–96. http://doi.org/10.1038/nature14232

35. Claus, S. P., Guillou, H., & Ellero-Simatos, S. (2016). The gut microbiota: A major player in the toxicity of environmental pollutants? *Npj Biofilms and Microbiomes, 2*(1). doi:10.1038/npjbiofilms.2016.3

36. Lai, K., Chung, Y., Li, R., Wan, H., & Wong, C. K. (2016). Bisphenol A alters gut microbiome: Comparative metagenomics analysis. *Environmental Pollution, 218*: 923-930. doi:10.1016/j.envpol.2016.08.039

37. Potera, C. (2015). POPs and gut microbiota: Dietary exposure alters ratio of bacterial species. *Environmental Health Perspectives, 123*(7): A187. http://doi.org/10.1289/ehp.123-A187

38. Choi, J. J., Eum, S. Y., Rampersaud, E., Daunert, S., Abreu, M. T., & Toborek, M. (2013). Exercise attenuates PCB-induced changes in the mouse gut microbiome. *Environmental Health Perspectives, 121*(6): 725–730. http://doi.org/10.1289/ehp.1306534

39. Zhang, L., et al. (2015). Persistent organic pollutants modify gut microbiota–host metabolic homeostasis in mice through aryl hydrocarbon receptor activation. *Environmental Health Perspectives, 123*(7): 679–688. http://doi.org/10.1289/ehp.1409055

40. Claus, S. P., Guillou, H., & Ellero-Simatos, S. (2016). The gut microbiota: A major player in the toxicity of environmental pollutants? *Npj Biofilms and Microbiomes, 2*(1). doi:10.1038/npjbiofilms.2016.3

41. Potera, C. (2014). Clues to arsenic's toxicity: Microbiome alterations in the mouse gut. *Environmental Health Perspectives, 122*(3): A82. http://doi.org/10.1289/ehp.122-A82

42. Lu, K., et al. (2014). Arsenic exposure perturbs the gut microbiome and its metabolic profile in mice: An integrated metagenomics and metabolomics analysis. *Environmental Health Perspectives, 122*(3): 284–291. http://doi.org/10.1289/ehp.1307429

43. Salim, S. Y., Kaplan, G. G., & Madsen, K. L. (2014). Air pollution effects on the gut microbiota: A link between exposure and

inflammatory disease. *Gut Microbes*, *5*(2): 215–219. http://doi. org/10.4161/gmic.27251

44. Sagar, N. M., Cree, I. A., Covington, J. A., & Arasaradnam, R. P. (2015). The interplay of the gut microbiome, bile acids, and volatile organic compounds. *Gastroenterology Research and Practice, 2015*: 1-6. doi:10.1155/2015/398585

45. Braniste, V., et al. (2014). The gut microbiota influences blood-brain barrier permeability in mice. *Science Translational Medicine*, *6*(263): 263ra158. http://doi.org/10.1126/scitranslmed.3009759

46. Carpenter, S. (2012). That gut feeling. *PsycEXTRA Dataset, 43*(8). doi:10.1037/e609662012-015

47. Yunes, R., et al. (2016). GABA production and structure of gadB/gadC genes in lactobacillus and bifidobacterium strains from human microbiota. *Anaerobe, 42*: 197-204. doi:10.1016/j. anaerobe.2016.10.011

48. Abautret-Daly, Dempsey, E., Parra-Blanco, A., Medina, C., & Harkin, A. (2017). Gut–brain actions underlying comorbid anxiety and depression associated with inflammatory bowel disease. *Acta Neuropsychiatrica,* 1-22. doi:10.1017/neu.2017.3

49. Cenit, M. C., Nuevo, I. C., Codoñer-Franch, P., Dinan, T. G., & Sanz, Y. (2017). Gut microbiota and attention deficit hyperactivity disorder: New perspectives for a challenging condition. *European Child & Adolescent Psychiatry.* doi:10.1007/s00787-017-0969-z

50. Petra, A. I., Panagiotidou, S., Hatziagelaki, E., Stewart, J. M., Conti, P., & Theoharides, T. C. (2015). Gut-microbiota-brain axis and effect on neuropsychiatric disorders with suspected immune dysregulation. *Clinical Therapeutics*, *37*(5): 984–995. http://doi.org/10.1016/j. clinthera.2015.04.002

51. Ibid.

52. Preterre, C., et al. (2015). Optimizing western blots for the detection of endogenous α-synuclein in the enteric nervous system. *Journal of Parkinsons Disease, 5*(4): 765-772. doi:10.3233/jpd-150670

53. Mulak, A., & Bonaz, B. (2015). Brain-gut-microbiota axis in Parkinson's disease. *World Journal of Gastroenterology, 21*(37): 10609–10620. http://doi.org/10.3748/wjg.v21.i37.10609

54. Rao, M., & Gershon, M. D. (2016). The bowel and beyond: The enteric nervous system in neurological disorders. *Nature Reviews. Gastroenterology & Hepatology, 13*(9): 517–528. http://doi.org/10.1038/nrgastro.2016.107

55. Ibid.

56. Rehfeld, J. F. (2015). Gastrointestinal hormone research – with a Scandinavian annotation. *Scandinavian Journal of Gastroenterology*, 1-12. doi:10.3109/00365521.2015.1025831

57. Rea, K., Dinan, T. G., & Cryan, J. F. (2016). The microbiome: A key regulator of stress and neuroinflammation. *Neurobiology of Stress, 4*: 23–33. http://doi.org/10.1016/j.ynstr.2016.03.001

58. Kelly, J. R., et al. (2015). Breaking down the barriers: The gut microbiome, intestinal permeability, and stress-related psychiatric disorders. *Frontiers in Cellular Neuroscience, 9*: 392. http://doi.org/10.3389/fncel.2015.00392

59. Mori, K., Nakagawa, Y., & Ozaki, H. (2012). Does the gut microbiota trigger Hashimoto's thyroiditis? *Discovery Medicine,* 14(78): 321-326.

60. Zhou, L., et al. (2014). Gut microbe analysis between hyperthyroid and healthy individuals. *Current Microbiology, 69*(5): 675-680. doi:10.1007/s00284-014-0640-6

61. Guo, Y., et al. (2016). Association between polycystic ovary syndrome and gut microbiota. *PLoS ONE, 11*(4): e0153196. http://doi.org/10.1371/journal.pone.0153196

62. John, G.K., & Mullin, G.E. (2016). The gut microbiome and obesity. *Current Oncology Reports, 18*(7): 45. doi: 10.1007/s11912-016-0528-7

63. Wouw, M. V., Schellekens, H., Dinan, T. G., & Cryan, J. F. (2017). Microbiota-gut-brain axis: Modulator of host metabolism and appetite. *The Journal of Nutrition, 147*(5): 727-745. doi:10.3945/jn.116.240481

64. Stress. (n.d.). Retrieved August 04, 2017, from https://www.merriam-webster.com/dictionary/stress

65. Dunckley, V. L. (2012, November 17). Screens and the Stress Response. Retrieved August 04, 2017, from https://www.psychologytoday.com/blog/mental-wealth/201211/screens-and-the-stress-response

66. Sturniolo, G. C., Leo, V. D., Ferronato, A., D'Odorico, A., & D'Incà, R. (2001). Zinc supplementation tightens "leaky gut" in Crohn's disease. *Inflammatory Bowel Diseases, 7*(2): 94-98. doi:10.1097/00054725-200105000-00003

67. Ahmed, S. H., Guillem, K., & Vandaele, Y. (2013). Sugar addiction. *Current Opinion in Clinical Nutrition and Metabolic Care, 16*(4): 434-439. doi:10.1097/mco.0b013e328361c8b8

68. Avena, N. M., Rada, P., & Hoebcl, B. G. (2008). Evidence for sugar addiction: Behavioral and neurochemical effects of intermittent, excessive sugar intake. *Neuroscience and Biobehavioral Reviews, 32*(1): 20–39. http://doi.org/10.1016/j.neubiorev.2007.04.019

69. Rippe, J., & Angelopoulos, T. (2016). Relationship between added sugars consumption and chronic disease risk factors: Current understanding. *Nutrients, 8*(11): 697. doi:10.3390/nu8110697

70. De la Monte, S. M. (2014). Type 3 diabetes is sporadic Alzheimer's disease: mini-review. *European Neuropsychopharmacology : The Journal of the European College of Neuropsychopharmacology, 24*(12): 1954–1960. http://doi.org/10.1016/j.euroneuro.2014.06.008

71. Added Sugar in the Diet. (2017, March 03). Retrieved August 04, 2017, from https://www.hsph.harvard.edu/nutritionsource/carbohydrates/added-sugar-in-the-diet/

72. Steele, E. M., et al. (2016). Ultra-processed foods and added sugars in the US diet: Evidence from a nationally representative cross-sectional study. *BMJ Open, 6*(3). doi:10.1136/bmjopen-2015-009892

73. Credit Suisse Research Institute. (2013). Sugar: Consumption at a crossroads. Retrieved from wphna.org/wp-content/uploads/2014/01/13-09_Credit_Suisse_Sugar_crossroads.pdf

74. Uittamo, J., et al. (2011). Xylitol inhibits carcinogenic acetaldehyde production by candida species. *International Journal of Cancer, 129*(8): 2038-2041. doi:10.1002/ijc.25844

75. Choudhary, A. K., & Lee, Y. Y. (2017). Neurophysiological symptoms and aspartame: What is the connection? *Nutritional Neuroscience,* 1-11. doi:10.1080/1028415x.2017.1288340

76. Paolini, M., Vivarelli, F., Sapone, A., & Canistro, D. (2016). Aspartame, a bittersweet pill. *Carcinogenesis.* doi:10.1093/carcin/bgw025

77. What is Celiac Disease? (n.d.). Retrieved August 04, 2017, from https://celiac.org/celiac-disease/understanding-celiac-disease-2/what-is-celiac-disease/

78. Fasano, A., Sapone, A., Zevallos, V., & Schuppan, D. (2015). Nonceliac gluten sensitivity. *Gastroenterology, 148*(6): 1195-1204. doi:10.1053/j.gastro.2014.12.049

79. Mansueto, P., Seidita, A., D'Alcamo, A., & Carroccio, A. (2014). Non-celiac gluten sensitivity: Literature review. *Journal of the American College of Nutrition, 33*(1): 39-54. doi: 10.1080/07315724.2014.869996

80. Drago, S., et al. (2006). Gliadin, zonulin and gut permeability: Effects on celiac and non-celiac intestinal mucosa and intestinal

cell lines. *Scandinavian Journal of Gastroenterology, 41*(4): 408-419. doi:10.1080/00365520500235334

81. Lammers, K. M., et al. (2008). Gliadin induces an increase in intestinal permeability and zonulin release by binding to the chemokine receptor CXCR3. *Gastroenterology, 135*(1): 194–204.e3. http://doi.org/10.1053/j.gastro.2008.03.023

82. De Punder, K., & Pruimboom, L. (2013). The dietary intake of wheat and other cereal grains and their role in inflammation. *Nutrients, 5*(3): 771–787. http://doi.org/10.3390/nu5030771

83. Ibid.

84. Fasano, A. (2012). Zonulin, regulation of tight junctions, and autoimmune diseases. *Annals of the New York Academy of Sciences, 1258*(1): 25–33. http://doi.org/10.1111/j.1749-6632.2012.06538.x

85. Jönsson, T., et al. (2006). A Paleolithic diet confers higher insulin sensitivity, lower C-reactive protein and lower blood pressure than a cereal-based diet in domestic pigs. *Nutrition & Metabolism, 3*: 39. http://doi.org/10.1186/1743-7075-3-39

86. Frassetto, L. A., et al. (2009). Metabolic and physiologic improvements from consuming a Paleolithic, hunter-gatherer type diet. *European Journal of Clinical Nutrition, 63*(8): 947-955. doi:10.1038/ejcn.2009.4

87. Zhu, W., Yang, J., Wang, Z., Wang, C., Liu, Y., & Zhang, L. (2016). Rapid determination of 88 veterinary drug residues in milk using automated TurborFlow online clean-up mode coupled to liquid chromatography-tandem mass spectrometry. *Talanta, 148*: 401-411. doi:10.1016/j.talanta.2015.10.037

88. Pal, S., Woodford, K., Kukuljan, S., & Ho, S. (2015). Milk intolerance, beta-casein and lactose. *Nutrients, 7*(9): 7285–7297. http://doi.org/10.3390/nu7095339

89. Merras-Salmio, L., et al. (2014). Markers of gut mucosal inflammation and cow's milk specific immunoglobulins in non-IgE

cow's milk allergy. *Clinical and Translational Allergy*, 4: 8. http://doi.org/10.1186/2045-7022-4-8

90. Haug, A., Høstmark, A. T., & Harstad, O. M. (2007). Bovine milk in human nutrition: A review. *Lipids in Health and Disease*, 6: 25. http://doi.org/10.1186/1476-511X-6-25

91. Daley, C. A., Abbott, A., Doyle, P. S., Nader, G. A., & Larson, S. (2010). A review of fatty acid profiles and antioxidant content in grass-fed and grain-fed beef. *Nutrition Journal*, 9: 10. http://doi.org/10.1186/1475-2891-9-10

92. Publications, I. O. (n.d.). Meet real free-range eggs - real food. Retrieved August 04, 2017, from http://www.motherearthnews.com/real-food/free-range-eggs-zmaz07onzgoe

93. Foran, J. A., Carpenter, D. O., Hamilton, M. C., Knuth, B. A., & Schwager, S. J. (2005). Risk-based consumption advice for farmed atlantic and wild pacific salmon contaminated with dioxins and dioxin-like compounds. *Environmental Health Perspectives*, 113(5): 552–556. http://doi.org/10.1289/ehp.7626

94. Sprague, M., Dick, J. R., & Tocher, D. R. (2016). Impact of sustainable feeds on omega-3 long-chain fatty acid levels in farmed Atlantic salmon, 2006–2015. *Scientific Reports*, 6: 21892. http://doi.org/10.1038/srep21892

95. Mccance, R. A., Sheldon, W., & Widdowson, E. M. (1934). Bone and vegetable broth. *Archives of Disease in Childhood*, 9(52): 251-258. doi:10.1136/adc.9.52.251

96. Koutroubakis, I. E., et al. (2003). Serum laminin and collagen IV in inflammatory bowel disease. *Journal of Clinical Pathology*, 56(11): 817–820.

97. Frasca, G., Cardile, V., Puglia, C., Bonina, C., & Bonina, F. (2012). Gelatin tannate reduces the proinflammatory effects of lipopolysaccharide in human intestinal epithelial cells. *Clinical and*

Experimental Gastroenterology, *5*: 61–67. http://doi.org/10.2147/CEG.S28792

98. Patisaul, H. B., & Jefferson, W. (2010). The pros and cons of phytoestrogens. *Frontiers in Neuroendocrinology*, *31*(4): 400–419. http://doi.org/10.1016/j.yfrne.2010.03.003

99. Rasnik et al. (2017). Influence of diet on the gut microbiome and implications for human health. *Journal of Translational Medicine*, 15:73. https://doi.org/10.1186/s12967-017-1175-y

100. Kotler, B. M., Kerstetter, J. E., & Insogna, K. L. (2013). Claudins, dietary milk proteins, and intestinal barrier regulation. *Nutrition Reviews*, *71*(1): 60-65. doi:10.1111/j.1753-4887.2012.00549.x

101. Hering, N. A., et al. (2011). Transforming growth factor-ß, a whey protein component, strengthens the intestinal barrier by upregulating claudin-4 in HT-29/B6 cells. *Journal of Nutrition*, *141*(5), 783-789. doi:10.3945/jn.110.137588

102. Magge, S., & Lembo, A. (2012). Low-FODMAP diet for treatment of irritable bowel syndrome. *Gastroenterology & Hepatology*, *8*(11): 739–745.

103. Ramadass, B., Dokladny, K., Moseley, P. L., Patel, Y. R., & Lin, H. C. (2010). Sucrose co-administration reduces the toxic effect of lectin on gut permeability and intestinal bacterial colonization. *Digestive Diseases and Sciences*, *55*(10): 2778-2784. doi:10.1007/s10620-010-1359-2

104. Ramdath, D., Renwick, S., & Duncan, A. M. (2016). The role of pulses in the dietary management of diabetes. *Canadian Journal of Diabetes*, *40*(4): 355-363. doi:10.1016/j.jcjd.2016.05.015

105. Kim, et al. (2016). The effects of dietary pulse consumption on body weight: A systematic review and meta-analysis of randomized controlled trials. *American Journal of Clinical Nutrition*, *103*(5): 1213-1223. doi:10.3945/ajcn.115.124677

106. Jayalath, V. H., et al. (2014). Effect of dietary pulses on blood pressure: A systematic review and meta-analysis of controlled feeding trials. *American Journal of Hypertension, 27*(1): 56–64. http://doi.org/10.1093/ajh/hpt155

107. Karkle, E. N., & Beleia, A. (2010). Effect of soaking and cooking on phytate concentration, minerals, and texture of food-type soybeans. *Ciência e Tecnologia de Alimentos, 30*(4): 1056-1060. doi:10.1590/s0101-20612010000400034

108. Gibson, R.S., Yeudall, F., Drost, N., Mtitimuni, B., & Cullinan, T. (1998). Dietary interventions to prevent zinc deficiency. *American Journal of Clinical Nutrition,* 68(2 Suppl): 484S-487S.

109. Tang, D., Dong, Y., Ren, H., Li, L., & He, C. (2014). A review of phytochemistry, metabolite changes, and medicinal uses of the common food mung bean and its sprouts (*Vigna radiata*). *Chemistry Central Journal,* 8: 4. http://doi.org/10.1186/1752-153X-8-4

110. Ros, E. (2010). Health benefits of nut consumption. *Nutrients, 2*(7): 652–682. http://doi.org/10.3390/nu2070652

111. Ibid.

112. Wu, F., Stacy, S. L., & Kensler, T. W. (2013). Global risk assessment of aflatoxins in maize and peanuts: Are regulatory standards adequately protective? *Toxicological Sciences, 135*(1): 251–259. http://doi.org/10.1093/toxsci/kft132

113. Bayman, P., Baker, J.L., & Mahoney, N.E. (2002). Aspergillus on tree nuts: Incidence and associations. *Mycopathologia, 155*(3):161-9.

114. Tournas, V., Niazi, N., & Kohn, J. (2015). Fungal presence in selected tree nuts and dried fruits. *Microbiology Insights, 8*: 1–6. http://doi.org/10.4137/MBI.S24308

115. Tamang, J. P., Shin, D.-H., Jung, S.-J., & Chae, S.-W. (2016). Functional properties of microorganisms in fermented foods. *Frontiers in Microbiology, 7*: 578. http://doi.org/10.3389/fmicb.2016.00578

116. Ibid.

117. Mota, A. C., Castro, R. D., Oliveira, J. D., & Lima, E. D. (2015). Antifungal activity of apple cider vinegar on candida species involved in denture stomatitis. *Journal of Prosthodontics, 24*(4): 296-302. doi:10.1111/jopr.12207

118. Sarkar, D., Jung, M. K., & Wang, H. J. (2015). Alcohol and the immune system. *Alcohol Research : Current Reviews, 37*(2): 153–155.

www.ingramcontent.com/pod-product-compliance
Lightning Source LLC
Chambersburg PA
CBHW071324210326
41597CB00015B/1335